Feed Your Real Hunger

Getting off the Emotional Treadmill that Keeps You Overweight

You can do it!

Jill K Thomas

Cover Art: Jennifer Kelly-Matthieu

Editing: Chris Zook & Kimberly Koga

ISBN# 978-0-9847054-0-5

Jill Thomas is not a physician or psychotherapist. The ideas, meditations and suggestions in this book are not intended as a substitute for medical or psychiatric care. Consult your medical professional on all issues relation to your mental and physical health.

Thank you to my hypnotherapist Michele Meiche who helped me find my purpose.

And to my husband Richard who helped me bring this book to life.

Most especially thank you to all the clients who have shared their stories and their lives with me these past years. I feel truly blessed to have known you.

Contents

Introduction: The Secret to Losing Weight

What is the secret to losing weight? *Eat less calories than you burn in your daily activities.* Not really a secret is it? In fact, by now there are probably very few people on the planet who don't know that. Armed with that simple information, why aren't we all at our ideal weights instead of taking part in this unprecedented health/obesity epidemic? Two reasons: 1) it is difficult for people to reverse a lifelong habit of overeating and 2) overeating is just a small part of the story of why someone is overweight. The real question to ask is "Why aren't we able to do what we need to do in order to achieve optimal health for the rest of our lives?" For most people this question isn't easy to answer, however it is the key to truly understanding our challenges with weight.

Knowing what you know about how to lose weight, how many times have you tried to lose weight and failed? how many times have you blamed yourself for failing to lose weight? "I can't stick to a diet because I have no self-control." "I can't seem to stop eating; I like food too much." "I am so fat, yet I just want to eat all the time." Have you ever considered that maybe the diet itself is not the problem? Perhaps there are bigger issues keeping you from being able to follow a given diet and do the things you need to do in order to lose weight? There may be reasons beyond simple self-control that make losing weight and keeping it off permanently, using diet and exercise alone, nearly impossible.

Most weight-loss programs put you on a diet and exercise routine, teach you tricks on how to burn more calories, and have you eat lots of low-cal, low-fat food, much of which you wouldn't normally eat. Basically these programs work on weight loss from the neck down focusing on the physical aspects, and almost always failing to achieve permanent success.

Why don't typical diet and exercise programs create long-term success? The truth is you didn't fail; you just tried to solve the wrong problem. The problem you really needed to solve is the one in your mind. It's the activity from the neck up that controls every action you take or don't take. It's what makes cake sound really good when your plan is to "watch what you eat," and exercise sound like torture after you decided to add it to your morning routine. It's the initiator behind everything, and if for one reason or another it doesn't want to lose weight and keep it off, you will never fully succeed, causing yourself nothing but upset and frustration.

Being overweight is not the problem—it is a symptom of a problem. The problem is that we have created an unbalanced relationship with food, a relationship that not only makes us fat, but will also kill many of us prematurely in one way or another. Since it's the fat and not the underlying emotional issues that we see every time we look in the mirror, we think it's about self-control. Rather than the fact we are fat because we have unhappiness in our lives, unhealed wounds, or other non-physical reasons why we feel driven to eat more than we need. So we try to fix it with diet and exercise. And sometimes that works for a while, and then we have trouble following our diets, become discouraged and depressed, which in turn causes us to overeat and gain back all the weight we lost, plus more, all the while feeling like we failed.

So, again, in spite of the fact we all know what to do in order to lose weight and be the healthiest version of ourselves, why aren't we doing it? Because, (for reasons I will discuss later) we don't *feel* like it, so we end up fighting against ourselves to lose a few pounds that we almost always gain back, typically with a few extra. In the process, we create habits that keep us overweight and keep us from succeeding at our ultimate long-term goals.

Think of a habit as being similar to a groove on a vinyl record album. The needle will continue to follow its predesigned groove and come out with the same result (song) every time. By shifting your habits, you are actually recording new grooves that are more in line with your current goal of losing weight so that the new habits become automatic and thus a permanent part of your life. Some say it takes 21 days create a new habit. I like to round it up to an even 30. That 30 days of conscious effort can change a non-life-affirming habit, like emotional eating, where you get upset and reach for food, to a positive, more life-affirming habit, like reaching for your journal when you get upset.

In some ways this might sound easy, but it can be very hard. As you will learn later in this book, there are reasons why we do the things we do, and those reasons create blocks that lock those negative habits in place and resist our attempts to change them. This book will help you get past those blocks and old ways of being so that you can create positive and lasting change. You will encounter some resistance however; this book will provide you with tools to help you move past that as well.

It Starts in the Mind

If it's really our thoughts and feelings that control what and how much we eat, it makes sense to start with the mind, right? So why don't we? Because we have been led to believe that the only reason we are overweight is because we are not on the right diet or exercise routine. This has come from our cultures obsession with physical beauty which has led to us demand help from the scientific community whose role is to explain weight gain from a verifiable physical perspective not an emotional one. Another reason this approach has become so prevalent is that there is no product to be sold (beyond a book or two) by telling potential clients the problem is really in your head. There's simply no money to be made by honestly stating, "You can go on a diet, but the results won't last if you don't get your head fixed." Such a statement would render moot an entire multibillion dollar industry that sells vitamins, diet programs, diet food, exercise equipment, and gym memberships, based on the premise that your weight problem is solved by investing in something outside of yourself.

However, the biggest reason we don't start with the mind is because in a lot of ways, it's much more difficult to deal with. For example, we have difficulty understanding why we want to eat more food than we need, why we constantly sabotage our own best weight-loss efforts, and why we wouldn't want to do every single thing we could to be absolutely healthy forever. After all, a pint of Ice Crème every night isn't worth giving up bathing suits for life, is it? So why do we do it? That's a harder question to answer than "Which diet should I chose?" because getting the answer involves really looking at our feelings in order to gain an understanding as to why we "love" things like French fries so much when they can so greatly interfere with our goals of creating a lifetime of optimal health.

Years ago I figured out how to deal with the underlying reasons why I was overweight and I used these principles to end a near-lifelong weight problem. I lost 75 pounds in a single year without going on any special diet, without doing extreme amounts of exercise, or taking weight-loss pills of any kind. And once I addressed the core reasons why I was overweight, doing the things I needed to reach my ideal weight became less of a struggle and more automatic. I did change the way I ate, and I did exercise more, but once all parts of my personality, including the "inner saboteur," were engaged in helping me achieve my goal, those changes came without struggle.

This program is about getting to the heart of the problem that causes you to eat more food than you need and to feel like exercise is painful. Those underlying issues usually hit you on a feeling level: "I crave chocolate." "I didn't feel like working out." For most, the *feelings* always speak much louder than your rational mind, which would say: "I like chocolate, but it's not as healthy for me so I will pass." Or, "I would rather sleep in, but it's better for me if I get my workout in early so I will do that instead."

This book will give you the tools you need to break down old non-life-affirming habits and behaviors and replace them with new ways of being that help you create the body and life you want. Most people in my Hypnotherapy practice tell me that by using this program, they were able to maintain their losses, and they felt like they had better control. People also tell me that their urgent feelings for food, sugary foods in particular, were greatly diminished. Usually at the end of a "diet program," people go off the diet and return to the old habits that created their problem in the first place and the weight quickly comes back. However, by starting with the more subtle issues of the mind, this program ends with you adopting new "thin person" habits that you keep forever.

In addition to focusing on the mental changes, I also include tips on physical changes you can make once you have addressed all the whys of the behaviors that got you into this position. But perhaps the most important tool in this book is meditation, which can help you retrain your unconscious mind to create more life-affirming habits. These are all tools I used both on myself and with clients to lose weight and to improve overall health and wellness.

As you quickly discover, this program is unlike any you have ever done before. It's not a diet. It's not an exercise routine. It's a mental shift that enables you to address those real underlying reasons you are overweight so that you automatically do the things you need to do so you can lose weight without the struggle or self-sabotage. This book asks you to go deeper and actually examine your emotions around eating, look at any reasons why you might actually want to be overweight, and consider how overeating is serving you in your life so that you can find other ways to meet those needs.

Not everything in this book will resonate with every person, and if something doesn't feel right for you, it's important that you honor yourself and not bring it into your life. However, I would encourage you to consider all the ideas presented and then set aside the ones that don't fit in your life.

Before we begin our journey, I will share with you my personal challenges with weight and how I came to write this book.

My Story

I wasn't always overweight. As a young child I was very healthy, active, and very skinny. Family albums from my early childhood are full of pictures of me running, playing, and being happy. Later on in life, I was grateful for those early pictures because they were proof that at one point, things had been different. But in spite of these external appearances, my family life was not happy.

My father had an angry, sometimes violent, temper that was often directed at me. It seemed to erupt without warning and, at times, without cause. If he wasn't hitting me for something I did, he was yelling or acting like a bully. The harsh words he would use were often worse than the hitting, because, unlike a bruise I could point to and blame my dad for, the demeaning and critical words stayed with me, and I took them as truth, leading to my low self-image and resulting weight problem. My mother called my dad's abusive behavior "discipline" and was unwilling or unable to keep me safe from the angry outbursts I was often the target of. I lived in fear for my physical safety for a large part of my childhood.

At some point early in my life I discovered the drug called *food* and used it for comfort, nurturing, and as a way to change how I felt anytime life didn't go the way I wanted, which for a child happens a lot. It became a crutch I used from my teen age years until about age 32 when I let go of being overweight forever.

Once I started puberty, hormones changed and my body matured. I then became fat, and that's where my near-lifelong struggle with weight began. As a child we moved around a lot, and I always seemed to be the fat kid in school in addition to often being the new kid. For this I was mercilessly teased by children at school and criticized by family who claimed they were worried about my health, though they actually seemed to be more concerned about how it looked to have an overweight daughter. As an adult, I developed even lower self-esteem, going through a series of bad relationships, some of them abusive, all the while feeling lucky to have those guys because I thought my weight made me unattractive. Those situations led to more and more eating and more and more weight gain until at my highest I weighed 220 pounds.

Some of you might be thinking "That's not much," and compared to the weight some people carry, it's not. But it doesn't matter how much you weigh, if it's more than is ideal for you, it can feel unbearable, and for me it was. I was in fact very active in sports and I so badly wanted my outer body to match up with all the effort and activity I put into making my body healthy and strong. So for me, being overweight became the single greatest issue I had in my life. I spent more mental energy, resources, and time trying to lose weight than I did on anything other aspect of my life—energy and time I could have spent improving my career, relationships, or anything else that would have made me happy. And because I didn't know any better, rather than trying to fix the real problem I had, which was an inner pain from a difficult childhood, I was going on diets and doing lots of exercise trying to heal the symptom of that problem—the fat.

Many of you can relate to the pain of someone saying, "She would be really pretty if she would just lose some weight," as I often heard from my brother's friends. Or having a co-worker tell me that my new boss, a former model only hired me because of my weight: "She is very insecure and wants women around her who she thinks aren't as pretty as she is." I actually laughed when I heard that even though it hurt. I couldn't help but respond, "At least for once being overweight helped me get a job."

"Well, if you were that miserable why didn't you just go on a diet?" you may ask. Oh, let me tell you about diets! I could write several books (and may someday) on all the different types of diets because, believe me, I have tried them all. Yes, *all of them,* and I have learned some very important things about diets and myself along the way. First of all, I hate cabbage soup, all meat diets make me feel very sick, all fruit or vegetable diets make me feel hungry all the time and cranky, 1,200 calories a day feels like starvation when you are used to 3,500- measuring and weighing is not something I am willing to do every day, and, most importantly, *diets don't work.* Nevertheless if you are reading this book, you have already figured that one out on your own.

"What about diet pills?" I have tried all those too, with the exception of the prescription ones Fenfluramine and Phentermine, commonly known as Fen-Phen, which got pulled from the market because of deadly side effects.

Instead I got so interested in vitamins for weight loss, and spent so much time studying and learning about vitamins, herbs, and natural hormone balancing, that I ended up working in the vitamin industry as a sales rep for almost 10 years. What I learned from working in that industry is that unless you have a deficiency or an imbalance in your system, vitamins alone will not make you lose weight; they are only a tool, you might see a small improvement, but only at great financial cost. Vitamins can help improve your overall health, wellness, and mood, which can indirectly help you lose weight but to date, I have found no vitamin or diet pill that actually results in permanent change.

"What about eating a more healthy diet?" It turns out that growing up, my family was vegetarian in a time before you could just go into any store and buy Garden Burgers and other healthy protein substitutes, so we, as a family, had to learn how to mix our grains to get complete proteins from our diets. Consequently, as a child I ate a very healthy diet with lots of fresh fruits and vegetables. I learned a lot about healthy eating and nutrition from my mom who had a passion for it. Eating healthy food wasn't ever really a problem for me. The problem was eating too much—*way too much*. And at an early age, I learned a very valuable lesson about eating: it's not just what you eat that causes you to be overweight it's how much. And what compelled me to overeat had absolutely nothing to do with food. It had to do with how I was using food and what purpose it had in my life and why I couldn't seem to get enough of it.

Rock Bottom

One of the lowest points of my life happened around the time I turned 30. I had been dating a man for over a year. We really weren't a good match, which was a source of great upset that caused me to overeat as a way of managing those feelings. During our time together my weight reached over 220 pounds, 20 of which I had gained while we were dating.

He wasn't a very nice person and would try to get me to lose weight by saying things like "No one is ever going to love you if you don't lose weight," and "Your friends aren't really good friends because they won't tell you the truth about how fat you have become." I felt lucky to have anyone so instead kicking him out of my life, I accepted his words as truth and allowed him to make me feel even worse about myself. The last straw came when he told me, "I'm sorry, Jill, but I just don't find you physically attractive, and I am not going to sleep with you again until you lose 15 pounds." I wish I could say I broke up with him right then, but like a deer in the headlights I just stood there stunned while he said the meanest words anyone had ever said to me in my whole life.

After I got over my shock, I called a friend who gave me some of the best advice I have ever heard. When I told her why I had to lose some weight for real this time, my friend said, "You stood there and let someone speak to you like that? Your problem goes much deeper than overeating. That deeper problem is what you need to address, not your weight." She was right, of course, and from that experience I learned that my weight problem was about more than just food; it was about self-esteem or lack thereof. In short, I saw very clearly I had a much bigger problem on my hands than an overpowering love for French fries.

Fittingly enough, this tragedy was followed by an inopportune photo opp. I was a hike leader for an outdoors club that posted pictures of all the leaders on their website. At my weight I looked huge compared to all the others and really stood out. Considering I was very active, it upset me that my outer body didn't seem to reflect all the exercise I was doing.

The last and most unfortunate convergence happened on the scale. It was my 30th birthday, and still newly single with eggs not getting any younger, I stepped on the scale and I will never forget seeing that glowing red number staring back at me 222 an all-time high. That number did me in, and I dissolved in a puddle of tears on my scale which I soothed with ice cream.

I've read articles in which drug addicts describe hitting rock bottom—that moment when it really hits them: what they have done to their families, their lives, their bodies, but, most importantly, to themselves. In a similar way, I can understand how it feels to hit the bottom of a very emotional situation. When I was at my lowest moment with my weight, I felt a great sense of despair and a feeling that I really did not want my life to continue in the way that it had been. I felt like I had dug a hole so deep in my life with my weight that I couldn't possibly climb out of it. And I knew it wasn't just my weight; it was my self-esteem, my personal dignity in letting someone into my life who would treat me poorly, and the even greater sense of knowing my weight did not represent what I was inside.

In my own mind, it felt like I had failed myself. I had let my body become something I was not happy with, but, more importantly, I didn't like feeling I was a slave to food. By that point, I knew that I was overeating because I was not happy with my life, I decided to reject that behavior. That day on that scale I made a decision: either I was going to find a way to make my body the healthiest weight it could be, or I was going to be happy with myself the way I was with no changes and grow my self-esteem from that place.

A girlfriend once told me, "The only time you make a vow that you actually keep is when you are upset," and she was right because on that day, I truly became free of my weight and feeling bad about my body. There was still a great deal to do and several twists and turns to my journey, but it all began with that day on the scale.

A New Beginning

Just after my breakdown I began to think about how much money, time, emotional energy, self-blame, and sadness I had been investing in my life as a fat person, and it really made me sick. I was beating myself up about the problem. I decided I was going to quit dealing with all the upset over my weight, and I was simply going to find a way to make it OK and accept myself just as I was with no changes. Basically, I was giving up on the joyless process of diet and exercise that I was repeating over and over again.

Something very magical happens when you give up and let go of something that you are really sick of: you open up space in your life for something else to come in. After I had made that decision, I heard the intuitive voice in my head say, "It didn't work because you were doing it all wrong." I have tapped into my inner intuitive information throughout my life, and usually the messages are subtle, like a whisper in my mind, but this time it was yelling at me, as though it had been trying to give me this information all along and I hadn't been listening.

I realized that rather than trying to control my food, I should eat what I wanted and learn to listen more to my body's own messages about what I should eat and how much. This completely flew in the face of my "1,200-calorie-a-day of low-fat foods with a side of two hours of exercise" model. Exercise was important, but I needed to take a more holistic approach that incorporated my lifestyle and things I enjoy doing rather than the boot camp-style workouts I kept trying to make myself want to go to but would always find a reason not to.

To my logical mind, these ideas made no sense; after all, doesn't spin class burn more calories than yoga? But my inner voice kept reminding me, "Yes, but you never go to spin class, so it doesn't matter how many calories it burns." That was true. I love yoga, and the bike does nothing for me; yet, I had been trying to force myself to go to spin class with no success. What about food? How am I ever going to control myself since I love food so very much? "Yes, but trying to *control* what you eat has never worked either." Very true. I can honestly say up until that point I had never been able to stick to a diet for more than a few months, even with many modifications. And truthfully, with the exception of the Atkins Diet, I was never able to stay on it for more than a few days.

Once I started to listen to my inner guidance, new ideas began flowing into my head and I also began to connect with new as well as new people who had different ideas about how to lose weight. Some of these new weight loss ideas were hard for the logical part of my mind to believe since they were so different from what I had been taught in the past; yet, I had nothing to lose as nothing else had worked.

As part of my personal weight-loss journey, I enlisted the help of an amazing hypnotherapist, Michele Meiche. With her help, and the use of hypnosis, I was able to address the underlying reasons why I was holding on to the weight and to free myself of fat-creating habits so that I could keep the weight off forever. I found these techniques so beneficial that I eventually decided to become a hypnotherapist myself in order to show others how to use these tools.

One year and 75 pounds later, which I've kept off for five years, I am very grateful I had the courage to try a different way of getting to my most ideal weight.
Let me share a few things I wish someone had told me before I started the process of losing all that excess weight.

Ten Things You Will Never Find in a Weight Loss Brochure:

1. Losing weight is one of the hardest yet most rewarding things you will ever do for yourself. Anyone who tells you otherwise is trying to sell you something.

2. After you lose over 40 pounds, you will probably have to buy clothes from the skin out (meaning you will have to replace underwear and bra's too) and that will cost more than you think, so start saving now.

3. There are people in your life, some very close to you, who will not want you to succeed and may even try to interfere, and this can be very upsetting.

4. When you lose a lot of weight, your whole life changes, not just your dress size, and some of

the people currently in your life may fall away, but that will be OK.

5. To lose weight you may have to face what you most fear: dating and being the center of attention. Being looked at in a sexual way can be very uncomfortable if you have spent a long time feeling like "the fat person," which can make you feel almost invisible.

6. Your body may be thin, but that doesn't mean your mind will think like a thin person until you make that shift on the inside.

7. People will treat you differently once you are thinner. Sometimes that will be good, and other times that will take some getting used to. (We'll work on that later, too.)

8. When you are fat, you think to yourself, "If I were only thin, I would be happy." Unfortunately being thin does not automatically make you happy; you still have to find happiness within yourself.

9. There is nothing you will gain as a thin person that you couldn't have had as a fat person, and when you really see that, you might feel mad at yourself for letting that weight hold you back from having the things you wanted a long time ago.

10. Just as eating donuts does not make you gain weight overnight, the positive changes you make won't cause you to lose it overnight either. Losing weight takes time and effort. Give yourself the time it takes to create lasting success.

Making Lasting Weight Loss Changes

In order for changes in weight to become permanent, the impetus for it can't be just about having a lower number appear when you step on the scale. Losing weight sounds good, but it will only make some parts of you happy, and that won't get all parts of your personality fully engaged in creating lasting change. The part of you that likes to be creative needs to get as excited as the part of you that wants to wear a bikini. You need to help your "whole you" to create a state of optimal health in your mind, body, and spirit. For this to happen, you need to be able to rediscover and become more comfortable with your real inner self and heal those parts of you that have suffered past hurts, find things that bring you joy, and connect with your higher self—whatever that is for you. Then you need to become aware of the negative eating and exercise behaviors you currently do automatically. Awareness is the key to everything. You can't resolve something unless you are able to truly become aware and understand it at several levels.

Through a series of exercises and guided meditations, this program is going to help you see the reasons behind your behaviors, taking your actions out of the realm of the unconscious and into the conscious mind so you can really deal with what's been driving your weight issues all along. We spend so much of our day paying attention to the outer world, we forget to look within and examine how we really feel inside. It's important to do this because it's those inner mental states and feelings that drive the behaviors that cause your body to be fat or thin. Also, when the mind is calm and relaxed we can more easily access the internal programming of the unconscious mind that generates our habits, and in turn change those automatic behaviors into ones that will help us achieve our highest goals.

Your unconscious mind doesn't know the difference between a real or imagined event. This is why, when you wake up from a nightmare your heart is pounding and you feel scared. If your unconscious mind knew it wasn't real, this wouldn't happen. Since your unconscious mind is where your habits are generated, it's important to connect with it through meditation and to feed it the imagery that you would like to create for yourself - that is more in line -

with your goals. For example, by feeding your unconscious mind images of a thinner person living a thinner person's life, you are telling part of you that creates your habits, "This is what I am now so I need to create habits that match this way of being." Over time and repeated efforts, your unconscious mind will start developing new habits that are consistent with that new lifestyle and you will automatically start eating less and working out more. By contrast, one reason so many people who actually hit their goal weight gain it all back so quickly is because on the unconscious level they think/feel like they are still fat. So when the diet ends, and all the control goes away, but the habits of the unconscious mind were never changed so they revert back to the same "overweight person" they are in their mind.

Meditation 101

The meditative state of mind feels a lot like the dreamy way you feel when you first wake up and when you begin to fall asleep—the mind is very relaxed and aware while your body is not yet active. This is because the brain waves your mind uses at those times put you in a semi-hypnotic state. Like in the dream state, the rational part of your mind that doesn't believe certain things are possible (like flying without a plane) slows down, enabling you to see and feel that all things are possible, including things that are otherwise blocked from your fully conscious mind. In this state you can move past any preconceived ideas, prejudices, or programming that you've created as a defense mechanism.

You have probably already experienced the meditative state it many times without knowing it. For example, ever notice how when you are doing something you really love, the world feels like it just fades away and you lose all sense of time? That is the meditative state.

I have been meditating as part of my religious practice since I was a young child, but until I started working on creating optimal health for myself, I hadn't used that tool for achieving a specific goal. As an adult, I discovered that guided imagery, which when done in a meditative state, is an amazing tool for life transformation and a way of creating both inner peace and lasting change. There are many ways of getting into the meditative state. For those of you who are new to the practice I suggest you use the following technique as a way of practicing this process. You will also be using it to help you deepen the meditations later in this book.

Deepening the Process

To get into a meditative state, start by finding an area in your home where you can sit and relax undisturbed for a while. You may find that quiet classical music helps you relax, like Chopin's nocturnes. Then close your eyes and shift your attention and focus to the inside by becoming aware of the ebb and flow of your breath. You will gradually become aware of thoughts, word pictures and ideas flowing around inside you. Just notice them and let them be there. Do this for a few moments.

Now notice that just below all that mental noise is a quiet stillness and go into that stillness. Imagine yourself going down a staircase deeper and deeper into that place of stillness, peace and quiet. And while you may still hear noise, focus your attention on the feelings of peace. See that the feelings of peace coming in waves and allow each wave that to bring you even deeper inside. Enjoy that stillness as long as you like, and when you are ready to come back, open your eyes bringing that feeling of refreshment with you into your life.

How to Use This Book

This book is broken up into a series of lessons. Some will take a week or longer; others will take only a couple of days. Work at your own pace, and allow all the information to really sink in before moving on to the next section. Some of the ideas on losing weight will be vastly different from the ones you grew up believing, and if something doesn't sit right with you personally, then perhaps that section doesn't apply to you, and that's ok-everyone is different. However, the ideas we grew up believing about how to lose weight were either completely untrue or not the whole story, I ask you to really try to openly consider everything I say before deciding it's not for you. I highly recommend that you do each section in the order presented as each section builds on the one before it.

This can be an emotional journey, so you will want to keep a private journal to track your progress and record any insights and understandings as well as concerns and frustrations so that when you are done you can see how far you have come.

Are you ready? Great! Let's get started.

Lesson 1: What Are You? Hint: It's Not Your Weight

What are you? That is a very philosophical question, and each and every person needs to find the answer within themselves. However, sometimes it's easier to find out what you are not. You are not your body, your body type, your clothes, your dress size, and, most especially, you are not your weight.

Your body is the vehicle you use to express yourself in the world; it in no way reflects the higher self which is your true nature. Your weight is really just a lighted number that stares up at you from a glowing digital metal plate when you stand on it in the morning. The same thing goes for your clothing size: it's just a gauge, a somewhat inaccurate one I might add, to help you determine which clothes are most likely to fit you when you try them on. You are not the store you buy your clothes in either, whether it's designer, department, or plus size; those are just the places you go to find clothing that fits your lifestyle, body size, and tastes. And you are certainly not your percentage of body fat. That is just another number you and your doctor use to measure your level of risk for certain health problems. Having said all of that, for the purposes of this book, it's important to stress again you are not your body or your weight.

This is a very important distinction, because so many of us are strongly identified with our current weight, and as being someone who is overweight that it can be hard to imagine our life any other way. It becomes as much a part of us as our name and our hometown. Words and thoughts have power, and if we keep reminding ourselves we are a certain size or weight, we start to become very attached to that body type and what we think it means to be that way. As a result, we match our thoughts, words, and actions to what we think an "overweight person" would do. We don't try on bikinis, we don't apply for jobs we think an overweight person wouldn't get, and we don't attempt to form friendships or romantic connections with people we think wouldn't be friends with someone overweight.

When I ask clients what they would like help with, I hear a lot of them say, "I am here because I'm fat," as though they are literally a ball of fat rather than a person who has a situation in their lives that they would like help changing.

I know for myself, this was a major problem. I so identified myself as being a fat person and with my body size that I almost saw it as part of my innermost self. For example, whenever I entered a room full of strangers, I would gravitate to the heaviest people like we were all part of a special club. It felt safer that way, but it was also very limiting. Because I, like many people, felt on some level that overweight people were inferior, I would not reach out and take risks that would get me ahead as I feared it would only result in failure. This was true in almost all areas of my life, including romantic relationships, personal relationships, and in my job in sales. For example, even though I was very qualified and had the skills to be a great outside sales rep, which paid very well, I always applied for jobs in inside sales (which paid less) because I felt very uncomfortable with my appearance and didn't want to meet clients face to face. In seeking relationships, even just friendships, I didn't approach people who seemed prettier or healthier than me, even though sometimes those were the people I really needed to connect with in order to grow as a person. Basically, I let my weight define me and hold me back. Not because I really was inferior, but because I let myself believe I was because of my weight.

The feeling of inferiority about my weight was the most challenging and the most important issue I had to overcome. The process of overcoming it helped me not only lose weight, but live my life to the fullest and appreciate myself more.

It's very important that you see what you really are. You are a person with all the wonderful things that go along with that. You are special and unique with qualities that no one else on the planet has in exactly the same way.

You have the power to create, destroy, love, hate, forgive, and influence lives, and your life has a special purpose that only you were meant to fulfill. Yet knowing all that, many people choose to identify themselves as "fat" rather than as someone who is worthwhile and working toward creating the most optimal health for themselves. This seems very sad, and what I most hope my book helps to heal.

Being over your most ideal weight, no matter how much over that number you are, is not a flaw, it's just a situation, perhaps one you are working on changing. Shifting the identification from the body to the situation enables you to remove the emotional aspect. Many of my clients find it so difficult to talk about how painful it is to be overweight that they have a hard time being clear about the simple facts of their physical health. In some ways the emotions make the problem seem much bigger than it really is. And these layers and layers of upset around being overweight are like glue holding the weight in place. The more you tap into how you feel about it, the more you want to eat and the bigger that problem becomes.

Society in general loves labels. Ask any child about their friends, and you will hear things like "That's Bob; he's smart," or "That's Tom; he's tall" It's human nature to want to boil things down as much as possible so we don't take up a lot of space in our brains with too much information. Nevertheless labels can be very detrimental because they cause us to place the sum total of our personal characteristics into one tiny cubby hole (in this case "fat"). And not only is that small "fat" cubby hole a tight squeeze, it's very hard to get out of.

We also judge others severely or extra pounds no matter how much we weigh. Have you ever caught yourself thinking, "I may be overweight, but at least I am not that bad. How could she let herself go like that?" Not a very nice way to think about someone who may only be 20 pounds heavier than you and might even have a medical condition that got her there. Since we judge ourselves so harshly for our own weight, we often project our inner self-loathing onto others. It's human nature to want to feel superior to someone else, especially if we were already feeling depressed about our own weight. In any case that judgment of yourself and others can really interfere with your goals.

Did you know that a few hundred years ago being overweight was very fashionable? And it still is in some cultures. It's often regarded as a sign of being affluent enough to eat large amounts. Being thin meant you were poor and likely of a lower class. Ah, the good old days! Regardless, most health care practitioners would agree that having a lower weight will greatly contribute to living a longer, happier, and healthier life - and that is a good thing. I can tell you from personal experience, it feels pretty freaking good to be at a healthy weight, and I wouldn't trade it for all the cake in the world. But as I've said before, that didn't happen for me until I stopped identifying myself with my body type and started seeing it as merely a situation I wanted to change and a challenge I wanted to overcome.

Its important to note that separating out the feelings does not make those emotions go away or heal all the hurts from your past experiences. That work has to be done separately. In the coming chapters, I will show you how to work on the emotional/feeling side of your weight issue. In any case, for now it's very important that you just start realizing that there is the problem, and then there is the story and the emotional aspect of the problem. Most of the story, the idea that being fat makes you bad, is a lie as are the feelings that result from that lie. The key is to start acknowledging that these ideas are lies.

Exercise: What You Really Are

Thinking of yourself as a weight, body type, or dress size is a habit, and, just like any habit, it can be changed. You need to start by creating a list of positive things that exemplify your true nature-the things you really are. Create a list of at least 10 positive things about yourself. These are going to be your new truths that I want you to remind yourself of when you start to think you are a certain body type, size, or weight. Here are some qualities that may apply to you:

I am smart.
I am funny.
I am pretty.
I am a good business woman.
I am a good mother/wife.
I am a good swimmer.
I am a good communicator.
I am a good problem solver.
I am very good at creating systems.
I am loving and fun.
I have a nice personality.
My body is in good shape.

It's important that you list what you feel good about, but not compared with others. For example, compared to a professional athlete you may not be considered a good swimmer; however, if you swim well and feel good about it, write it down.

Now the very next time you think "I am so fat" or "I can't believe I weigh ___," I want you to stop and tell yourself at least three things on your list. They must be positive and uplifting. We will get into this more in the section on the power of words, but this is just to get you started. Of course, you aren't going to make your mind stop thinking those thoughts; that would be impossible and would probably drive you crazy (ask me how I know this). I recommend you watch yourself for the next 30 days to create that new habit of shifting your identity from something negative to something positive. I know it seems impossible now, but if you do this, you really will start to look at your weight more objectively and less personally, and that is a big key to losing weight.

Meditation: I Am Not My Weight

Sit and relax quietly and focus your attention on your breath. Notice the ebb and flow of each breath and allow your inhalation to bring in peace, relaxation and comfort while you allow each exhalation to help you relax more deeply inside. Now begin to find that place of inner nothingness using the deepening process from earlier in the book to more fully relax into it.

When you are ready, picture yourself not as a body, but as a giant being of energy, as light. Imagine that light growing brighter and stronger. Now seeing yourself simply as energy, step out of your body for a moment and imagine yourself floating through your life, observing your family and friends and activities—feeling free of restrictions, social expectations, and physical limitations - free to be whatever you want to be. Allow yourself to really enjoy that feeling of being free.

While enjoying this relaxed state, ask yourself what changes you would like to make. For Example:

- How would you be in a world free of the ideas about what you are?
- What would you really like to be doing now that you are free of limitations?
- What would you like to improve?
- How would you like to grow as a person?

Now become more aware of your body and notice that, just like a piece of clay can be molded and changed, you have the power to change your body—know that physical bodies can change and become healthier and that it's possible to change yours to be more ideal.

You decide that you would like your body to become the healthiest version of yourself and be aware that just by thinking it, your body begins to change, and soon you are able to see and feel yourself at your ideal weight. Feel yourself being surrounded by your most ideal body. See it as changeable and flexible and healthy. Then observe yourself walking around in your healthiest body, going about your day experiencing your life from that place and becoming more and more comfortable. Continue to visualize yourself moving around in your ideal body until it feels very natural, even more so than the one you used to occupy.

When you feel yourself fully connected with the healthiest version of your body, allow yourself to return to the world and enjoy this new state of being.

Now spend some time writing in a journal about what you observed and learned from this meditation and what changes, if any, you decided to make in your body and life. In the next section, you will use that information to help you create goals for yourself and formulate a solid image of what your new body and life will be.

Summary

Remember that first and foremost, you are not your weight, and you are free to make any changes you want, but all of that starts by acknowledging that your true self is far greater than any number on the scale.

Lesson 2: What Do You Want and Why?

It's very hard to accomplish anything substantial in life without a clear idea of exactly what you want, why you want it and how your life will be improved by making this change. So the first step in any journey is setting a goal. In this lesson, I want you to make some decisions. I want you to spend some time deciding exactly what you want to get out of this program, what your health and weight goals are, and what you want your life to be like as a result of creating optimal health. To that end, ask yourself the following questions:

What do you want to do that you think you can't do now? Things like taking a long hike without running out of breath, buying clothing off the rack, etc.

What life experiences do you want to have that you feel you can't have now? Things like feeling comfortable in a bathing suit out in public or dating if you feel that your weight is holding you back in this area.

What do you want to weigh? If you chose a goal weight, make sure it's realistic. I tell my clients to be flexible about their weight and chose a number that excites them, but be open to the idea that when they hit their ideal size, it might not be that weight. It's not as easy as simply looking at a chart. Everybody is different, so don't get too attached to a specific number; it may be more or even less. Once you get there you will know.

What size do you want to be? I suggest you make a size your main goal unless that doesn't excite you. If you exercise a lot or are more muscular, your size could be heavier than someone else's. I know from experience that a size 10 can be 130–155 pounds or more.

What do you want to look like? With this one, it's very important you create a realistic picture in your mind of your ideal appearance. It must be something you are physically capable of achieving. Every single person is different, and you can't just pick a picture from a magazine and tape your face over it. "I want to look like Heidi Klum." Me too, actually, she's beautiful! But with Photoshop, many of the magazine pictures make the model appear smaller than she really is. And if you are someone with a larger frame, it may not be physically possible for you to ever be as small as those women in the magazines. On some level your mind knows this, so if you are a larger framed woman and you decide Lindsey Lohan's body is your ideal, your mind will say "Yeah, right!" and you won't feel like it's even possible.

If you're like me and have never been your ideal size, and thus have no real picture of what that should look like, find someone in your life to emulate. There was a trainer at my gym that, like me had a larger, stockier body. One day I asked her what she weighed and her size. Though I think she found the question strange, she did tell me she weighed 155 and wore a size 10. That really helped me get motivated, because at least I had an idea what I would really be looking forward to.

You should now create a list of at least five clear goals for yourself so you know where you are going.

The next part of this is to get a very clear *why* you want to achieve these goals. Think about "What is the payoff?" "What's in this for me?" As human beings we don't do anything unless we get something out of it. For some, that payoff might be feeling healthier and stronger or experiencing feeling thin or whatever else most excites you. If you have a strong motivating reason or payoff for creating optimal health, then that reason will keep you going when the process becomes difficult—and trust me on this one, it will get difficult at times.

Also, the goals and the "whys" have to be for you personally. Often I see clients who want to lose weight because they want the approval of others as in: "My husband really wants me to lose weight," or "My kids/doctor/sister, etc., are concerned about my health." For these people the journey can be more difficult because, though they may genuinely want to lose weight, it's hard to achieve something if the motivation is about pleasing someone else rather than themselves. This *has* to be about what you want. So often, we do things in life because we seek love, approval, and, most importantly, acceptance from others. But those motivations will not get you through the rough times on this journey and keep you inspired when its 6 a.m., raining, and you don't want to go work out.

The last part of this is to find a way to have at least some of what you are hoping to accomplish before you actually achieve your weight-loss goals. So many people put things that are important to themselves on hold because they think we have to have the perfect body first. At this time it seems like a form of punishment to wait until you have lost weight before you do kind things for yourself, like dressing in nice clothing or to begin dating again.

If you weigh 300 pounds, you may not be able to climb a tall mountain right now, but you can certainly enjoy a nice nature trail in the woods. Why wait for something you really want when you can have some part of it now?

Here are some examples of how you can bring a part of your goals into your life now:

Goal: *"I want to be able to go into the petite section of the store and buy a nice size 10 summer dress that I can wear to a party."*

You can have that now by going to a nice plus-sized store and picking out a nice outfit that makes you look and feel amazing. Many of the major department stores are also now offering their best fashions in larger sizes.

Goal: *"I want to be able to say "no" to the office donuts on Friday just because I can."*

Maybe saying "no" would be too hard at first, but perhaps you could just have half of a donut or bring your own dessert snack that's healthier than the donut. Or, since one donut is usually not enough to kill your diet, just plan on having a smaller breakfast and lunch and enjoy the donut.

Another more advanced version of this approach is to practice taking back your power and saying "no" to one particular food item every day so you get a feel for it. As you practice this more and more, it becomes easier. Try picturing yourself at your ideal weight when you are offered a donut. Then decide if you would rather have the donut or a healthier body. It's easier when you can actually see the healthier body in your mind.

Goal: *"I want to be able to wear a flattering swimsuit at the beach."*

The truth is you can wear one now, but since what you really want is to have a nice, healthy looking body, I would recommend you go to a store that specializes in bathing suits and ask a professional to help you choose one that minimizes your trouble spots and enhances the nice curves a fuller figure gives you. A well-fitting and nicely shaped suit can make a huge difference in how you look, no matter how much you weigh.

Goal: *"I want to look nice so I can go out on dates."*

I have asked a lot of men the question, "What do you find most sexy in a woman?" The most common answer is "confidence," followed closely by "a sense of humor" not a size 2 body, though I will admit I have heard that. Find a way to feel confident and good about yourself now, no matter your size, and then you will attract more of the kind of attention you are looking for. Or, if it's the nice date you want, dress up and take yourself out on one, and invite a friend to go with you. The company will be great, and you will be able to do whatever you want. The more you allow yourself to feel special now, the easier it will be to create that special feeling in a relationship.

Often what happens is we use what I call the "weight excuse" as the reason why we don't give ourselves what we really want in life. We may even feel like it's pointless to spend money on nice clothes or to create better health for ourselves at the weight we are now. However, that idea that we're not good enough, just as we are, is one of the things that can drive us to eat more than we need in the first place. To wait until we are "thinner" before we give ourselves things we want feels a lot like punishment for being fat and it will not help us succeed long term.

Try on Your New Body—New Life

The other reason why it's so important to practice giving yourself at least some of what you want now is that in order for your new body and new weight-loss habits to take hold, your life as a "thin person" has to feel as comfortable and as close to the norm as possible; otherwise, it won't feel enough like you to stick. In a way, you have to practice trying on that new life every day so that *the new life and new body* feel more comfortable than being in the old overweight body. The following meditation will help, I recommend doing it often.

Meditation: Step into a New Body

Now that you have a clear picture of what your new body and life will be like, and why you want it, it's extremely important that you practice trying it on regularly. Start with every day for the first 21 days and, after that at least two times a week. Since this meditation very important, I have included it as a free download on my website. Visit www.feedyourrealhunger.com to download the "Weight loss" daily meditation.

Allow yourself to relax, close your eyes and begin focus your attention on the ebb and flow of your breath. Use *the deepening process* from earlier in the book to become very comfortable and deeply focused on the inside.

See yourself in your bedroom preparing for your day, deciding how to do your hair and what you are going to wear. As you get ready, become aware of the fact that there is a part of you that has already achieved your health and weight-loss goals; this trimmer inner self has already done what it takes to reach your goals and already knows what life will be like from the place of being thinner and healthier.

Call this part forward now and see your healthier inner self standing in front of you. Notice what's different. Notice how you will look at your ideal weight, how your clothing will fit, and how your face will look. Now I want you to step into that ideal body, almost as though you were stepping into a piece of clothing. Feel yourself moving around in your ideal body. Notice how your clothing feels and how much physically stronger you feel at your ideal weight.

Now observe yourself going about your day as your thinner self. Notice that you have different habits. See yourself automatically choosing healthier food, getting more exercise, and feeling more energized and freer now that you have lost the extra fat and have achieved your highest goals. Notice the other differences, too. Take note of how much more confident you feel, how much healthier and better you feel about yourself and your body. Take a moment to allow yourself to really appreciate the differences.

Decide that today you are going to wear your inner healthier body and spend your day feeling and acting as though you had already achieved your goals. Really anchor that body around you so that you really feel your new healthier self on your outer body. When you feel yourself fully merged with your healthiest body and able to live life today from that place, go ahead and open your eyes and begin your day as your healthiest self.

After having done this meditation and focused on being your thinner self while in a relaxed state, did you notice anything different about what you thought you wanted on the outside and what the thinner self appeared to be on the inside? How did it feel to be your thinner self? Did it look/feel differently than you expected it to? Make note of how you felt in your weight-loss journal and notice if those feelings change as you practice this meditation more. Don't be surprised if you notice a lot more details as you go along.

Summary

The more you practice trying on your thinner body, the more it will feel like you. Since your unconscious mind doesn't know the difference between what is real and what is imagined, the more you tell it that this is the *real* you, the more likely it will be to match your unconsciously driven behaviors towards what someone at that ideal size would do. In other words, if your unconscious mind sees you as your thinner self, then it will shift your habits to be more in line with those of a thinner person, thus making it much easier to become that. And the more your behaviors match those of someone with the body you want, the faster you will have that body.

Lesson 3: Your Weekly Meeting

To achieve lasting success start thinking about the process of creating optimal health for yourself and liken it to a major project you have just been put in charge of at work. Like any project you do in your life, you have to have an objective, a plan, and the ability to adjust that plan as more information comes up or as things change and develop. To this end, I want you to schedule time on your calendar for a weekly Weight Loss Project Meeting. I recommend Monday because in the working world that's often when those types of meetings take place, but choose a date and time that works best for you. Every week I want you to do your weigh-in and sit down with yourself in an honest way and answer the following questions:

1) *What five things went well and according to plan this week?*
   You have to acknowledge yourself for all the little things that went well and according to plan, even if all you did correctly was the little things. The more you pay attention to the positive things, the more of those you will have.

2) *What three things did not go the way you wanted them to this week and why?*
   The "why" is very important because you have to understand what caused you to get off track and not stick to your plan? Be honest here: why didn't it work out? Is it because you don't like the exercises you chose to do, the diet you selected, or your goal was too ambitious? Whatever it was, you can adjust, but only if you are honest with yourself.

3) *Do you need to change the way you do things to make sure those three things get done in the best way possible next week?*
   No need to beat yourself up about anything. If you don't like something, you shouldn't force yourself to do it. For example, just find exercises you like, a healthy way of eating you can live with or any other adjustments you need to make to achieve success.

If you set aside time to work on your weight in this manner and are vigilant about it, you will start to really feel like this is a serious project and that you are serious about losing weight. On an unconscious level, a weekly check-in sends a powerful message to your inner self that you intend to succeed this time. It's very easy to get off track when you ignore what is going on in your life.

People often get so caught up in feeling like something "should" be working for them, and blaming themselves when it doesn't, that they forget to evaluate whether it really is. This is a long process and along the way you will have successes *and* failures, but it's essential that you always be supportive of yourself to keep the whole program on track.

I was once working with a client who had put herself on a very difficult diet and she was sure it would enable her to lose weight. After several weeks and no weight loss, this diet had only caused frustration. I looked over the diet schedule, and though it seemed complicated and restrictive, I determined that she could have lost weight. So I asked her, "Why do you think it didn't work?" "Well," she replied, "I kept cheating. If I only had more self-control, I could lose weight and this diet would work." She was right. This diet could work, but in reality it would never work if it's so hard to do that she couldn't stay on it. I explained to her that it wasn't her; the issue is the diet she chose did not really match her lifestyle and eating preferences. If she had sat down with herself in a non-judgmental way every week and really looked at this situation objectively, she probably would have seen this problem much earlier.

The best diet that will help anyone achieve optimal health is one that they can stay on long term. I will get into that more later, but for now just know if it's not something you could see yourself doing forever, it's not the right diet for you no matter how many celebrities supposedly lost weight doing it.

I know for myself, sitting down every week and doing an honest assessment of what worked and what didn't kept me on track and from losing interest throughout the process. In a way, I felt like I was really paying attention to my needs for the first time and making myself a priority, like being my own coach. If for some reason I hadn't lost weight, I would look at why, make changes if needed, and sometimes even determine that I needed additional help. I often consulted with a personal trainer who helped me keep my workouts hard enough to challenge myself but interesting enough to make it fun.

You have to put yourself first in this process, and making time for yourself every week is the first step.

Pay Yourself—The Game of Weight Loss

It can be hard to stay motivated and excited about something that can take a long time to achieve. For me it took almost a year to lose 75 pounds. Some weeks I lost three pounds, and some weeks I lost none.

Most of my life I have worked in sales, and in a lot of ways, the game of losing weight is like selling: sometimes you do everything right and perfect, but the sale never comes. Other times you show up late, make a bad joke at the meeting, discover the product you are pitching won't suit the customers' needs, and yet they buy it anyway for reasons that seem to defy logic. With my weight loss, I may have done my workouts for five straight days, passed up on 10 donuts brought in by coworkers, stuck to eating healthy 95% of the time, and still not lost a single pound. Other times I chowed down on pizza and chips with friends, consumed an unholy amount of calories, and still dropped a pound or two. Anyone who has watched the show *The Biggest Loser* has seen this too. They all work ridiculously hard, and sometimes they lose more weight than seems physically possible; other times, nothing.

Just as eating a donut does not automatically make your butt bigger, going for a jog in the morning will not make it smaller by the afternoon. It's all the little things done consistently over time that produce the results you want. As long as the overall trend is downward, and you are doing your work to make it happen, you are on the right track.

And here's another hard part: if you are over 200 pounds, even dropping 20 pounds may not change your appearance much, if any, and you might need to lose as many as 30 or 40 pounds before you drop a clothing size. I know this frustration very well. I probably lost 30 pounds before anyone noticed, and, even then, it was only my female friends. I was down almost 50 pounds before my dad said, "Jill, you are starting to look a little smaller. Have you lost some weight?" I actually thought he was kidding. He wasn't. He hadn't noticed because to him, I didn't look much different. By the way, for those of you women over 200 pounds, once you get down to the 170s, you only need to lose 5-10 pounds to go down a dress size rather than the 20 plus pounds you needed to lose at the higher weights. I happily discovered that one myself.

The trick I used to keep myself motivated was borrowed from my early days in sales. One of my first bosses would give us a bonus based on how many calls we made, knowing that that more calls would ultimately translate into sales. This kept us motivated in the beginning when there really wasn't a lot to show for our efforts. From this I learned it's important to reward yourself for both the effort and the results. So I would pay myself $2 for every trip to the gym and $5 for every pound I lost. I put the cash I "earned," which I had previously withdrawn from the bank, in a fish bowl so I could actually watch that pile get bigger as I got smaller. It was great motivation for me and a lot of fun. After returning home from my workout, I would grab a couple of crispy ones out of the bank envelope, and put them in the bowl. I loved it; it made me want to go more. Every Sunday I would step on the scale and pay myself $5 for every pound I lost. Some weeks I was putting in $15 for pounds and $6 for workouts; other weeks it was just $8 for workouts, and that was fine because I was still rewarding myself for the efforts that would ultimately produce the weight-loss results I wanted.

Though this is a fun and motivating way to stay on track, one thing I want to warn you: it's supposed to be about rewards and not punishing yourself in any way. *If for some reason you gain a pound, you are not to take back any reward from the bowl*. Self-punishment in any form just makes you feel bad, which causes you to eat more. Just start paying yourself again after you drop that one pound and then for the next one as well.

Another reason I don't want you to take money out when you gain some weight is because sometimes you will find you gain weight for reasons that make no sense at all. Women especially can gain and lose several pounds of water weight over the course of a day. I remember once going into my personal trainer's office crying and telling her that I had been doing everything right, yet I had gained three pounds. She didn't even look up from her desk and said, "It's been really hot lately, hasn't it?" Yes, it had been over 100 degrees almost every day that week. "I bet you have been drinking a lot more water, haven't you?" Yes, I felt like I had been drinking my weight in water that week. "Sometimes people retain more water when it's hot. Water equals weight. It will probably be gone by next week." She was right, of course. By the following week I had lost five pounds and learned a valuable lesson: a few pounds either way should never be that big of a deal for anyone.

If money is not how you want to reward yourself, then find a system that works for you, but make sure it's something you can touch and see building up and that you reward yourself for both the effort and the result.

Exercise: Preparing to Start Your Program

Schedule your very first weekly meeting on a day and time that will work for you every week. Monday may be too busy, but perhaps Sunday afternoon will always be free.

At this very first meeting, I want you to spend some time taking a real hard look at what did and didn't work for you in the past and why you think it failed. Be as honest as possible about what happened. It's true that almost all diets can help you to lose weight, but specifically what about your past approaches caused you to fail? Was it not enough food? Was it too different from the way you normally ate? Was it too time consuming to prepare a separate meal from the one your family was eating? Try to make your answers as specific as possible. Don't just say, "I did not have enough will power." Rather, be honest and say, for example, "I was hungry all the time on that diet."

Write down a diet or exercise routine you did in the past that failed in the long term. List what you liked, disliked, and something else you could do instead as a solution. Here are some examples from my own life:

The Atkins Diet
Dislike: worked for a while, but I wasn't able to keep it up long term. Didn't feel good when I was on it.
Like: loved that I could eat all I wanted of certain foods; that made me feel like I wasn't starving myself.
Possible solution: since I liked the "all you can eat" approach, perhaps looking into a similar low-carb diet would be good.

Boot Camp Class
Dislike: went for a while but found it hard to get up at 6 a.m. to go; sore all the time in the beginning and didn't really like it.
Like: I could really feel myself getting stronger; loved watching my muscles grow.
Possible solution: check into the 8 a.m. weight-training class instead.

Weight-Loss Diet Club
Dislike: found the food pricey and not very healthy; worked for a while but as soon as I went back to my old diet, I gained it all back.
Like: having someone to talk to every week about my progress and things I could do to succeed. Felt like I had a cheerleader.
Possible solution: there are some counseling programs like Weight Watchers that allow you to buy your own food. A nutritionist could also be a great help here.

Now from your list, think about how you might best lose the weight. Remember, it's all about you and on some level you already know what your body needs to achieve your weight loss goals, you just have to listen to that information. Later I will give you some strategies that will work, but for now it's important that you start getting ideas about what does and does not work for you personally and why.

Visit your doctor. If you haven't already done so, make an appointment to see your doctor and get a physical. It's good advice to consult your doctor before starting any weight-loss process. However, I am suggesting it not because this program is about doing lots of exercise (it's not), or going on a crazy diet (not that either), but because there are some very medical reasons why you may be having difficulty losing weight that are not going to be addressed in this book. For example I used to work at a hormone research lab, and I learned firsthand how hormone or vitamin/mineral imbalances, like having low iron or a thyroid problem, can really make it hard to lose weight no matter what you do, and I want you to rule out the possibility of a medical issue before you find yourself doing all the right things yet getting nowhere.

The other reason I want you to go is that it sends a message to yourself on both a conscious and unconscious level that you are serious about losing weight. Remember how buying new school clothes as a child would make you excited about going to school? Getting a physical and knowing where you are at physically is a very important preparation step for making your trip into optimal health. That way, in a year when you go back again, you will be able to see how many improvements you have made.

Visit a personal trainer. A personal trainer can check your body fat percentage and give you an idea of where you are with your cardiovascular health. Your doctor might do this as well if you request it. Personally, I prefer seeing a trainer for this because they have other tests for physical fitness that your doctor doesn't usually perform, such as a stretch test, balance tests, and a resting heart rate test, all of which will help you get a good idea of your overall physical condition.

From these appointments, you should get some idea of what a healthy weight for you would be and what percentage of body fat would be most ideal.

Weigh yourself. This one can be very scary since it means facing the truth about what has happened to your body. But weighing is not about beating yourself up; it's about being clear about where you are. To correctly weigh yourself, do it at the same time of day and only once a week. You may have already discovered that if you do it several times a day, your weight goes up and down a lot. Don't drive yourself crazy with this; it's just a number and not necessarily an accurate one. The bathroom scale is a gadget, not a self-esteem busting, torture tool.

Set up your reward system. As discussed above, having a visual reward system will bring you more of what you want. Seeing cash sitting in the jar next to my bathroom scale was one of the most motivating things for me when losing weight, and, trust me, I had to use every penny to buy new clothes.

But remember to make this fun. If it's enjoyable, you are much more likely to keep it up and ultimately succeed at this process. Love yourself enough to do what it takes to create the life you want.

After you have completed all of your preparations, do the following meditation to strengthen your commitment to this new path. This is a great one to do anytime you feel your resolve slipping.

Meditation: You Make the Choice

Allow yourself to relax and focus your attention inside. Use "the deepening process" from earlier to help you go a deep inside.

Now imagine yourself walking on a beautiful green path in the woods. It's a lovely day and the sun is coming in from behind the leaves. See yourself walking on a very clearly defined path. It's the path your life has been on, well worn and comfortable. It's the path that continues the current direction of your health and current body size. You know exactly where this is going, and you know where it has been.

Now see yourself coming to a fork in the road. On the left, the path continues as it has been, and it's very easy to follow since you know exactly how to continue that path. Now notice the path on the right. This path is curving upward and appears to be going in an entirely new direction, but it's currently covered in mist and fog, so you don't know exactly what that path looks like and what it will take to travel where it goes, but you are very clear on where that path will take you. It takes you to optimal health, a perfect-sized body, and a life of having all the things you want to gain from being free of the extra weight. It takes you to what you most desire and will bring you what you really want out of life. Imagine all those things you want as pictures or perhaps feelings or maybe even the words, whatever way comes easiest for you. Imagine what your life will be like once you get there, visualize pictures, feel the feelings and even hear the words of that new life. Know that this path, though somewhat unclear, will take you there.

Now bring into the picture of your crossroads two important parts of your personality. First, bring in the inner intuitive self, the part that helps you make important decisions and understand the deeper consequences of your actions. This part enables you to make choices that are in your best interests. Next, bring in your inner warrior. This is the part that makes you feel strong and safe and reminds you that all your choices will be OK and that you are always protected and loved no matter what you do. This part also gives you the courage to make hard choices in a way that sets aside the fear and brings in the light. Allow yourself to fully connect with these parts as you make the very important choice about which path to take. Know that either way is fine.

When you are ready to make your choice and walk down that path, whichever path you choose, fully commit to making this path a part of your life and feel happy with the choice you made. Now resolve to make all of your decisions from the place of being on this path, fully committed to doing what it takes to make that path a success.

When you feel yourself feeling happy and free about the choice you have made, open your eyes and resolve to do whatever it takes to commit to and be happy with that path for as long as it takes you.

Summary

Staying committed takes acknowledging what's real for you and how you want to lose weight, allowing failures of the past to be the past and moving into a new place. But mostly it's about committing to you. Love yourself enough to do what it takes.

Lesson 4: Clear out Your Closet

Goodwill charities used to run a radio ad that I really loved. It starts off at a support group meeting for weight loss and people are talking about how much they have lost on the "Goodwill Diet", and one man says he recently lost 240 lbs, another woman says she lost 50 Lbs. The suggestion of course being that getting rid of your old, unnecessary possession is a great way to lose weight of all that stuff. And it's so true on many levels! If you get rid of old things that are no longer serving you, or things that remind you of bad memories, you will lose weight.

I bring this up early in your transformational process because in order for you to bring something new into your life, you have to create space for it, both literally and figuratively. And what better way than to do it than by cleaning out the closets of your life. If you have read any self-help books in the last few years, you may have heard this advice before, but the way I recommend doing it takes this exercise to a new level, and every client of mine who has done this has lost weight, just from this one task.

Think of the items in your closet as pieces of energy: the energy it took for someone to create them, the energy it took you to earn the money to purchase them, and the energy required to maintain those things and the space they take up. In this way it's easier to see the stuff in your closet as stagnant energy, and letting those items go helps get that energy moving, allowing you to bring new things in—things that are more in line with what you currently want in your life, like smaller clothes to fit your new, healthier body and lifestyle.

As thinking and feeling beings, just looking at the objects in our closet brings up memories of pleasant or unpleasant events that make us feel good or bad about ourselves. Almost every woman who yo-yo diets keeps an assortment of clothing sizes as a way of reminding herself what size she *used* to be hoping that this will motivate her to work harder. Hint: that never works; those old thin-person clothes just make you feel bad and want to eat more. As part of the process of clearing space for something new, it's important that you not be assailed by memories of your weight-loss failures every time you open your closet.

I worked with a client who still had her wedding dress from 10 years ago hanging in her closet where she would see it every day. Not only was she no longer that size, but she had been divorced for two years! She had hoped seeing the dress would inspire her to lose weight so she could find a great guy and get married again; instead, that dress just made her sad. Letting go of it not only caused her to lose weight, but it helped her let go of a daily reminder of her failed marriage, and I am sure the woman who bought the dress at the thrift store was happy to have it.

I know when I did this exercise; the first thing I grabbed was a beautiful dress I had bought for myself five years earlier that I had never been able to wear. I had intentionally bought it smaller than my actual size to encourage myself to lose weight and stick to whatever diet I was on at the time. That diet, and the five or more that came after hadn't worked, so instead of being inspirational that very pretty dress hung in my closet as a constant reminder of my failure, and every time I saw it I felt bad, really bad. Feeling bad about myself did not motivate me to eat less; it caused me to run to my favorite thing for comfort: food. And it wasn't just that one dress. I had a full range of clothing in different sizes from one end of the closet to the other. It was actually a bit of work to figure out which clothes still fit.

If you knew your best friend was torturing him- or herself by constantly dwelling on past failures, you would intervene and encourage your friend to let that old stuff go, wouldn't you? Well, you are now going to be your own best friend and help yourself feel good about stepping in your closet again.

Exercise: Clean out Your Closets—All of Them

- Get rid of any clothing that is too small, too big, ill fitting, or *frumpy*—if you don't look good in it you won't feel good in it, so just let it go.

- Get rid of anything that reminds you of an ugly moment in your life: that shirt you wore the day you broke up with your boyfriend or girlfriend, old shoes that are too painful to wear, and, most especially, any wedding attire from failed marriages. You don't need to be reminded of that every time you open your closet.
- Go through your jewelry box and dresser and clear out anything that reminds you of a failed relationship or anything (like a bracelet or a watch) that doesn't fit or is broken. Take them to a "cash for gold" place, and turn that stuck energy into the unstuck energy of cash—then buy yourself something nice.
- Get rid of every piece of exercise equipment, including running shoes, that you haven't used recently or, even more common, ever used at all.
- Make sure you take down any *pictures* of yourself that don't make you feel good about your current body. This includes pictures of yourself at a thinner time if that is not where you are now.

The goal here is to be able to open your closet and see it full of things that fit well and don't remind you of ugly memories, look at your walls and see only pictures that make you happy, and see beautiful gifts you gave yourself out of love rather than a trinket from the ex you never liked. You don't have to throw these things away, but you do need to put them where you won't see them.

Symbolically, this process is about releasing the weight of those items and the memories, upsets, anger, or frustrations associated with those objects. Letting them go frees you of the energy those items possess, and the *weight* of those items will go with it. Love yourself enough to give yourself this gift of freedom.

Extending This Project into Your Life

Once you've cleared out your closets, extend the process into other areas of your life. For example, look at areas where resources, in terms of money, time, or energy, are going out to places that no longer make you happy and maybe never did. It's so easy to stay in a rut and continue to do what you always have done, but every once in a while, you really need to take a look at all the places your energy goes and reevaluate.

Time and energy: Create a list of things you expend energy on in the form of time: kids' soccer, volunteer activities, such as at church, clubs, and PTA, classes you are taking, etc. For each activity, ask yourself the following question: "Am I comfortable with the amount of energy in the form of time that is going out for this?" If yes, great; if no, it's time to make a change.

Money: Money is a very touchy subject, and one that causes people a great deal of upset, whether they have it or not. For the purpose of this exercise, I want you to consider that there may be things in your life you spend money on that really are not life affirming.

For one week, write down every penny in cash you spent and what it went to. Then gather bank statements and credit card receipts, and for each item or category of items ask the question: "Am I comfortable with the amount of time it took me to earn the money for that?" If you aren't, it's again time to make a change. If you haven't been to the gym in five years, perhaps it's time to either go or cancel that membership and use the money for something much more important.

Your mail: Opt out of any catalogs, magazines, and newspapers that you aren't really reading anymore. Stopping the catalogs is not only good for the environment, but it's good for your wallet too.
Unsubscribe to all the e-newsletters, blogs, and group lists that are just cluttering up your email inbox, i.e., you never open them. One of my clients spent 20 minutes opting out of all the e-newsletters she was getting and figured this saved her about two hours a week in time spent sorting through and dealing with unwanted emails.

This may not seem like it has a lot to do with losing weight, but trust me, the more you manage and pay attention to the ways you are spending your time and energy, the more you will be able to focus on what's really important—you!

Meditation: Letting go of the extra layers

Once you have gotten rid of all the extra stuff in your life and made sure you feel good about all the different ways you spend your time, money, and energy, it's time to do the following meditation to peel off the layers of extra fat and feel more comfortable being you. I do this with my clients, and it's a very powerful tool for change. Do it as often as you like.

Relax and focus your attention inside. Use the deepening process from earlier in the book to help you. Allow yourself to drift down even deeper than normal into your place of peace, the place where you go to reconnect with your true inner self.

When you are ready, imagine yourself walking on a lovely path through a beautiful meadow. It's a warm breezy day, and you are feeling very good inside. It's a very safe place, a place where you can truly be yourself. As you walk along this path feeling so relaxed and so much at peace, you start to feel a bit warm, and you decide to take off an extra layer of clothing that you have been wearing. It feels so good to let go of that layer that you decide to shed another, realizing that each time you shed a layer you become lighter and freer.

As you continue to walk along, you decide to let go of some of the fat that you have been carrying, allowing that fat to just melt away without effort and without fear. In the past you may have felt uncomfortable or even exposed letting go of that fat, but now you realize here in this magical space that it is completely safe for you to let go of the weight and be your most authentic thinner healthy self.

Still on the path, you continue becoming lighter and feeling healthier and more free to be yourself in this world. Since you know that eventually you will have to go into the outer world again, you decide to surround yourself with the most beautiful healing light of protection, choose the light that makes you feel most safe and free to be your real self.

Inside that light, you are protected, as the light and your logical mind keep you safe, so safe in fact that you are free to let go of the fat permanently and move around in the world without it.

Now that you have surrounded yourself with light and are completely safe, you start to imagine yourself in your outer world: your job, your home life, your friends, and all the places you go to do the things you do. As you think about this outer world, notice if there are any things you would like to change in order to make yourself feel even more safe and comfortable in that world.

In the past you may not have felt very comfortable in that outer world without a layer of fat, but because you have this new light-protection with you at all times, you are free to release the fat and be comfortable in your daily life being your real self. See yourself being very comfortable as your true healthy self out in world, feeling totally safe.

When you are ready, open your eyes to your new world, surrounded by light, feeling totally protected and safe.

Summary

Sometimes letting go of those old things that no longer serve you can be very emotional. Just know that it's OK to grieve over the memories, wishes, hopes, and dreams that haven't gone as you had planned. Just know that by clearing out the old, you make space for a more amazing future, one that will give you what you most want in life.

Lesson 5: Dismantling Beliefs

Now that you have cleared out the physical debris that was holding you back in life, it's time to look at the outdated beliefs that may be keeping you from reaching your highest goals. In this lesson we will be focusing on the beliefs you may have about losing weight and what it means to be fat—beliefs that are either completely untrue, not true for you anymore, or, more commonly, beliefs you picked up from others that no longer serve you and the life you want to lead.

I bring this up early in the process because this approach is so different from other programs out there. The old model for losing weight has been so ingrained in us that you may find yourself colliding with against outdated ideas regarding what will or won't help you lose weight. Those around you may find it hard to believe that working on managing your "feelings" and handling your emotions about food will actually help you lose weight. For many, the whole concept of examining how you feel about eating is just too touchy-feely when compared to more traditional approaches of going to the gym, dieting, or taking a weight-loss pills.

Beliefs are sticky things; we often think that we formed our opinions on our own. But when we really look at them, we often discover that these ideas came from family, friends, and/or society are simply untrue; yet, on an emotional level we still think they are real and live our lives accordingly. If you follow these old constructs about diet, food, and exercise, they really can hold you back, especially when you consider, as many of you have already discovered, that they don't work long term.

I am now going to ask you to examine many of those "truths" you hold about weight loss and to embrace some new ones. In short, I want you to keep an open mind and consider numerous and various ways of achieving optimal health. Some of these ideas you will like and use forever, others may not fit your lifestyle, if so you it's ok to can cast them aside. Not everything I say will apply to everyone nor will it all be every reader's personal truth, we are all on our own life path.

When you start to look at your life in general and examine your beliefs regarding health and wellness, something magical happens: you start to become more powerful.

Here are some ideas you may have been taught that are simply untrue or incomplete:

Old Idea: *You have to go on a diet to lose weight.*

Truth: To lose weight you do have to change your diet, but in only one way: eat less. However, to improve your overall health and increase your energy levels, you will need to make healthier food choices. The phrase "going on a diet" implies eating small amounts of low-cal foods for a little while then going back to your old way of eating. However, any form of short-term calorie restriction will not produce lasting results; for that you will need to permanently change your eating habits.

Old Idea: *You have to do lots of exercise to lose weight.*
Truth: Studies have shown time and time again that it's not the amount of exercise you do that determines your weight; it's how much you eat. However, exercise does improve your overall health and has a major impact on improving your mood. And when you feel happier and more confident, you make better choices. I have seen many clients get hung up on the idea that if they don't do rigorous exercises, they are never going to achieve optimal health, and that's simply not true. You can actually lose weight without exercising. So if you are someone with a physical limitation that makes exercise difficult, or you can't seem to get out of the house, you have just lost your excuse for not trying to improve your health.

Old Idea: *You have to give up all sweets to lose weight.*
Truth: Every nutritionist out there will cringe when I say this, but if you ate 1,200 calories of chocolate or potato chips and nothing else, you would lose weight. Now, that's only 4 candy bars (depending on which kind) or one big bag of chips, so I wouldn't recommend that approach. But it's important to be clear that it's the number of calories and not where those calories come from that determines how much you weigh.

Old Idea: *Being overweight means you have no self-control.*
Truth: Though this is a prevalent idea in our society, it's simply not true. If you really had no self-control, you would probably be in jail because you shot one of those

kids who teased you as a child and called you "fat." Know that "controlling" food doesn't help you lose weight, it actually makes things worse. Overweight people have just as much self-control as anyone in every other area of their life except this one. For them, it may feel a bit like being a drug addict or alcoholic but with food. Yet for someone who is not using food as a way of coping with life, it is very difficult to understand those feelings so, instead, they judge.

Old Idea: *"But losing weight is hard."*
Truth: Fighting yourself is hard. Beating yourself up for being "weak" is hard. Not being happy with yourself and your life is *really* hard. Dealing with weight-related health issues on a daily basis is hard. Not being able to have the life you want is extraordinarily hard. Yes, losing weight is hard, but it's so much easier than dealing with all those other things, especially when you stop fighting and start loving yourself through the process.

False Beliefs We Were Taught

There is another set of beliefs we picked up from childhood that are actually much more damaging than those regarding weight loss. They are false and limiting ideas about what or who we are as a person.

Take a look at any beliefs you have that start with "I am not _____ enough to…" followed with something you can't do. For example:

"I am not pretty enough to be a cheerleader."
"I am not smart enough to go to a good college."
"I am not tall enough to be a dancer."

These beliefs were often instilled in us by primary caregivers, such as our parents, babysitters, teachers and sports coaches, who hurled them at us during moments of anger and/or frustration. What makes them so damaging is that we always managed to confirm of their validity in our daily lives. "I am not attractive enough to get dates" is proven when you are turned down for a prom date by the person you are most attracted to at school - Your mind completely ignores the fact that you didn't want to go with that person anyway, or that they were already seeing someone. You may have also been able to prove "I'm not smart enough to go to a good school" when you were turned down by your first-choice college, completely ignoring the fact the school had a record number of applicants that year.

The other set of negative personal beliefs starts with "I don't deserve to be ..." and usually ends with happy, rich, thin, or whatever your mind fills in the blank with. Just know it's all nonsense.

You are *enough* for any of the things you want. You *deserve* all the best in life, and anyone who ever said otherwise is completely wrong. You can let go of those ideas that hold you back and allow yourself to move into a new and more wondrous place. Although it can be difficult to let some of these old beliefs go, it's essential to your weight-loss process that you drop the mental weight of those false ideas and the negative emotions they bring up. When you are ready, do the exercise later in this section.

Shifting Expectations

Years ago I dated a math professor at a local college. One day over lunch he posed a rather philosophical question to me about math. "So Jill, let's say you toss a coin 19 times and each time it comes up heads. What is the probability that on the 20th toss it will come up tails?" I had to think about it an embarrassingly long time before saying, "It's 50/50 right, just like the first toss?" "Yes, that's true and that's an obvious answer, isn't it? But you had to think about it?" I sure did, but I got his point. He explained that his students get stuck in that kind of thinking all the time. They look at the back story, the history, and try to create an outcome based on that rather than on the obvious facts. They, in a sense, are letting their feelings get in the way of their logical thought process. It seems logical to think that if the other 19 flips were heads, the last one would be too, but that's because you are basing your thinking on past experience. The coin itself doesn't think; it just does what you make it do. It's our mind that makes it mean something.

He was right, but I was struck by the bigger picture he was presenting here. We, as thinking, feeling beings do that all the time. We get stuck in our back stories. We allow our past experiences to determine our future success, so much so that we aren't even able to see the obvious answers right in front of us. In essence, we decide that we can or can't do something based on what happened before. This is often described as "baggage", but I think it's more accurate to say it's constructed expectations. In other words, we expect a certain result, so the mind starts to construct thoughts and ideas around that feeling, such as "not screwing it up this time," or how mad our partner will be if we spend a lot of money on a weight-loss program and it fails. In fact, we often approach many experiences with "I hope it works out this time," rather than expecting that it will, like you would if you were doing something you've have had past successes with.

Many of us, through countless attempts and failures at weight loss, have conditioned ourselves to start a process hoping for success, but on some level expecting it to fail. While I am not dismissing the fact you've failed in the past, I am saying that it means a lot less than you think it does. Today you have the power to change anything you want in your life. You can lose weight and keep it off forever, and that starts by confronting that feeling and not letting your past failures determine your future.

Exercise: Changing Your Beliefs

Now think about your ideas about weight loss and the truths you have been taught over the years. List as many of these beliefs as possible, paying special attention to the ideas that you have adopted that make you feel bad about yourself. I've listed some of the most common ones, but here are some more ideas about losing weight that you may have taken on that aren't true:

If I don't lose weight, I will never find true love.
If I don't lose weight, I will never get that great job
I have always wanted.
I am never going to be considered pretty if I don't
lose weight.
I can't wear a bikini if I don't lose weight.
I have to lose weight before this event or I will look
terrible.

**In addition, there are negative personal beliefs
like**:

I am not good enough to have what I want.
I have never succeeded before; why would I now?
I don't have enough self-control to stay on a diet.
I don't deserve to be happy.
I don't deserve to be healthy.

Next, I want you to analyze each of these ideas with
your logical mind and ask yourself "Are they really true?"
"Is there any tangible proof? Or did I, (or someone else)
just make them up. Am I using them now to beat myself
up?"

Also consider that these were once true for you
however, are they still true now? The reality is there will
always be certain jobs—like a TV news anchor, game show
host or model that may be nearly impossible to get if you
don't have a certain look. However, if there is some aspect
of that type of work you enjoy—like being in the public
eye—you can find a way to have it without being thin.
Oprah is the best example of this, although her weight yo-
yo'd over the years, she continued to attract some of t he
highest ratings on TV. People love her because she is
honest, open, and confident, and the same can be true for
you when you set aside limiting beliefs and let your true
self shine through. The point is to look at these "truths" you
have taken on to determine what's real and what's not.

Most false beliefs make no logical sense, yet we
continue to allow them to influence how we feel about
ourselves. Once we insert logic and reason into the

equation, we are able to more easily let go of these old ideas and make space for feelings and beliefs that will help us achieve our highest goals.

Once you have finished dismantling your list by looking at each item logically, I want you to create a new list of ideas and ways of being that are more in line with your true self and how you want to live your life. Include beliefs like:

> I can have anything I want.
> I can lose weight and still eat fun foods.
> I can be happy no matter how much I weigh.

After you have completed this exercise, do the following meditation.

Meditation: Burning Outdated Ideas

Allow yourself to get into a comfortable position. Use "the deepening process" from earlier in the book to relax even deeper. Now picture yourself on a beautiful beach at sunset enjoying watching the waves and feeling peaceful. Imagine a wonderful bonfire in this place where you start to feel warm and cozy as the fire grows larger.

Next to the bonfire is a stack of paper filled with words and ideas on them. These papers represent outdated or incorrect information you pulled from your own mind. Now see yourself throwing the words and ideas into the fire. Some of these ideas are untrue, some were never true, and some came to you from others, but now you are ready to let them go since they have been weighing you down for too long. As you toss each file onto the fire, really feel yourself being released from those ideas as though the ties to them are being released as well. See the fire consuming them and releasing them back into the nothingness from which they came.

Now that you are free of the old ideas, it's time to bring new truths into your life in a flexible way that will move you forward on your path. Begin by thinking about the new beliefs you wrote down in the previous exercise.

Be sure to include things like "I can have anything I want," "There is nothing stopping me from creating optimal health for myself," and "I can make any life change I want just by deciding to do it."

Feel yourself really accepting that new information and making it part of your life. Let the new ideas take hold and run the show for you, knowing that at any time you can release them when they become outdated.

When you are ready, open your eyes to this new way of being.

Summary

You have the power to decide what is true for you and how you want your life to be. Take that power back and chose to believe in things that make your life better rather than things that make you feel any less than your highest self. Again, it's your choice; decide to be happy and healthy and loving to yourself. Trust me; you will like the results of that choice.

Lesson 6: What Exercise Really Is

A couple years ago, the magazine *Time* published an article titled "Why Exercise Won't Make You Thin" (Aug. 9, 2009). The article explained what many health practitioners have been quietly saying for some time: Exercise alone will not make you thin; you have to actually change your diet. Now that we understand that exercise is not a tool for making you lose weight, we can consider its real value as a tool to enhance your health, happiness, and long-term well-being.

A personal trainer once told me a story that helped me see exercise's real value. Just after the birth of her second child, she had fallen into a deep depression which led her to see a doctor and ask for antidepressants. Her forward-thinking physician told her to go to the gym every day for 30 days and at the end of the month if she still needed the medication he would give it to her. It worked, she never went back for the drugs, and she came to love exercise so much that she decided to drop the 50 extra pounds she was carrying and become a personal trainer.

Exercise has to be something you do because you genuinely like it rather than something you do because you have to or else you are going to be fat and die a premature death. Having said that, I believe every person can find energetic activities that they like. Remember when you were a child and you felt the pure joy of running around in the yard chasing a ball? Now imagine if someone had taken that fun, unstructured play away from you and handed you a kettle ball and said, "Lift this 20 times over your head. Now switch hands. Now do 20 squats, 40 sit ups, and 20 pushups. OK, now that you are done, go sit in front of the TV for the rest of the weekend because you'll be too sore to do anything else." Would that have been any fun for you as a child? Probably not, and it doesn't do much for most adults either.

When exercise stopped being about play and started being a chore, we stopped liking it. Exercise has to be done in the spirit of play so that it brings you joy and helps you feel better about yourself as a person. If an early morning spin class is fun for you, then continue to do that, but if it isn't, find something you do like and make your time doing that exercise sacred. And don't get hung up on the idea that it has to look a certain way. I think four hours joyfully playing volleyball every Saturday is worth much more to you than boot camp classes that you hate so much you only go once a week even though you pay for three. There are so many energetic things you can do, why force yourself into something you don't like?

Below I've grouped the different types of exercises into three categories:

Contemplative exercises. These are exercises that allow and encourage you to think or zone out while your body works and moves. They include yoga, hiking, swimming, and solo jogging, where you can either contemplate your life stresses while you work your body and burn off those calories or you can drift into a meditative state and allow your body to really enjoy the movement, much like you would during a massage.

Social exercises. These are forms of exercise that can take place in a group setting, including team sports, jogging, hiking, dancing, or going to the gym with friends. The focus here is bonding through activities and working together in the spirit of play. One of the healthiest clients I ever worked with was on a rowing team. He mostly enjoyed the camaraderie of working as a team with his friends and the fact that it made him healthy was just a bonus.

Energetic exercises. Although all exercises can be energetic, some, like kickboxing, spin, running, or boot camp class, can emphasize pushing the individual to enhance the intensity or energy of the workout. These often result in a huge endorphin rush afterwards.

All of these types of exercise can make your body much healthier, improve your mood, and help you feel personal satisfaction. However it's important to remember to only choose ones that you actually like doing as opposed to ones you just think you *should* do. Don't force yourself into doing energetic exercises when you really want a slow, steady pace, and don't do more relaxing exercises when you are in the mood to get your butt kicked. Knowing what you want, doing what you want, and being flexible about choosing different exercises based on what you want that particular day is the way to lasting exercise success.

In this section we are going to explore how you can rediscover the spirit of play and find energetic physical activities that will make you happy. Most personal trainers I have talked to recommend 45 minutes of rigorous exercise three to four times a week. However, the reality is that if you try to force yourself to do something you don't like, you will end up doing *zero* minutes per week. So the trick is to find something you enjoy so much that you will want to do it on a regular basis. Use the following exercise to help you.

Exercise on Exercise

Begin by asking yourself the following questions:

- What physical activities do I really enjoy doing? (List at least five.)
- What activities have I always wanted to try but never have?
- How can I bring more of those activities into my life now?
- Where can I fit 40 minutes of exercise three or four times a week into my life?
- Who can I get to go with me?

This week, in addition to the above questions, take some time to list all the fun, play-type things that you like to do that involve some form of physical activity, no matter how mild that form is. Come up with at least five things that you find fun or new things that you would like to try. Often the local YMCA or community center will offer interesting classes that involve exercise, such as dancing, yoga, and Thai Chi.

Resolve to find a way to do one or more of these activities at least three to four hours a week, which should be fairly easy if it's something fun that you like doing. Try something new and explore different activities; you may find yourself discovering a new exercise that becomes a lifelong passion for you. The following meditation will help you reconnect with a love for exercise.

Meditation: Love to Exercise

Use the deepening process to become very comfortable and very deeply relaxed and focused on the inside.

As you get deeper into your relaxation, I want you to think about a time when you were doing something fun and energetic, some kind of exercise that brought you joy. Remember how it felt to move your body in an energizing and playful way. Perhaps you were running, or perhaps you were playing a sport. Really tap into those feelings of joy as you remember the activities you were doing. Now begin to think of at least three ways you can bring those same fun activities into your present life. Perhaps you can start jogging or join a sports league.

Now think about a time you did a more contemplative exercise like yoga, running alone, swimming, or hiking—any exercise that allowed you to feel peaceful while doing the activity. Really tap into the feelings of inner peace and mental focus that those activities engendered and think of three ways you can bring those activities into your life now. Perhaps take a yoga class or plan a hike.

Now think about a time you really enjoyed being with a group of friends doing exercise. Remember how much fun it was to feel like you were in it together on a team or bonding while playing a team sport like basketball, volleyball, or softball. Really feel how it felt. Then, think of at least three ways you can bring more of that into your life now. It could be just coming up with three friends to do exercise with, or it could be joining a sports league, whatever sounds like fun to you.

Next, imagine yourself choosing exercises that sound like fun and doing them. See yourself allowing the part of you that wants to exercise the freedom to choose what suits you best on any given day. See yourself fully supporting those choices, knowing it's the joy and fun that is most important.

When you feel very complete with this exercise, open your eyes to this new way of being.

In my experience there are few people who are able to sustain an exercise routine when the motivation is strictly about keeping the body fit. Exercise has to be something that brings you real satisfaction or you won't do it for very long. Again, don't be afraid to explore new and interesting activities.

Remember, it's about joy and play. Now go have fun!

Lesson 7: Portion Sizes and Calories

Counting Calories—Awareness Is the Key

Having just explained how exercise won't make you thin, but will make you happy, let's talk about something that will help you trim down: managing calories. I have always hated counting calories or measuring my portions. It just seemed like a ridiculous amount of work that I was usually only willing to do for about a day. The worst part for me was discovering how little food you can eat and still stay within the calorie restriction limits. It made me depressed, and I often binged the day after I started.

Counting calories always felt a bit like punishment for being fat, as I assumed that thin people never thought about calories. Having worked with many people who were what I considered "naturally thin," I discovered that most of them stayed that way because they do pay attention to the amount of food they eat. Though they may not necessarily count every calorie, they are aware of both the portion sizes and number of calories in the foods they eat every day so that they don't overdo it, which is very easy to do when you aren't paying attention.

When I first started my process of losing weight, I sought the advice of a personal trainer who suggested my old nemesis—counting calories. I of course objected because this had always been so hard for me in the past for a lot of reasons. Then she asked me a question that made me really rethink my feelings about calorie-counting. She said, "If you were to go into a department store, and you had $100 for a top and some jeans, do you think you could pick out an outfit that cost around that amount without looking at the price tags, just using your experience with how much things cost?" "Probably, if it was a store I shop in a lot, and I know what they usually charge." "OK," she said, "That's how you need to get with food. You need to train yourself to know, without looking it up, about how many calories are in the foods you are eating on a regular basis. It should be fairly easy since you probably eat the same things all the time, right?"

She was right. Like most people, I am a creature of habit and don't often eat lots of new foods. And if I did try something new, it was often just a variation of what I eat normally, like a chocolate milkshake rather than vanilla. What she said really convinced me that I should be aware of how many calories are in the foods I eat every day, not so that I can beat myself up about it like I have in the past, but so I can bring more awareness to my eating.

She suggested making a list of all the foods I normally eat with the portion sizes, and then calculating the calories for each. The key was to be so aware of how many calories were in the foods I ate on a regular basis so that I could just look at my plate and know if I am taking in a lot more than my body needed.

In a way it's a bit like planning a financial budget. Imagine if you were not paying attention to your money and were spending a $1,000 more per month than you were taking in? Unless you had a lot of savings, you would probably end up in some major trouble in a very short time. The same is true for calories. If you are not aware of how many calories are in the foods you eat, you could end up in very serious health trouble in a short time—some of you are already there. It's not about adding them up and getting upset. It's about knowing what's going on, so that you can adjust if you want and/or need to, and knowing what should stay and what should get reduced. You can't fix a problem unless you first understand it completely.

So how many calories should you eat? While I don't recommend making calories and calorie counting a huge focus, it's good to have some idea of what to aim for. My experience has been that the 1,200 calorie diets are way too hard for most people to stick to. Personal trainer Christine Burke of Light-Hearted Fitness has observed healthy weight management at 1,500-1,700 calories for women, depending on their exercise level, and 1,800-2,000 for men. She says it's typical for an overweight person to consume 3,000 plus calories per day.

Exercise: Calorie Awareness

1) **Buy a calorie counting book**. They make small ones you can fit in your purse or briefcase, and there are some great websites you can use to help you track everything.

2) **Pick a couple of typical eating days and start keeping track of your portion amounts**. Measure things. I know it's a pain, but when it comes to foods like cereal, I guarantee you are eating larger portions than you think you are. Pour the amount of cereal you would normally eat into a bowl and then into a measuring cup, and use the box to help you figure out the calories. Same thing with milk, coffee cream, butter, jam on your toast, dressing on your salad, and cheese in your taco. And don't assume because it's a "single-serving package" that it contains only one serving. Check the label on items like chips—often a small bag is actually two servings.

3) **Find better options for your heavy hitters**. Take particular note of the labels for foods you eat a lot that have lots of calories, like coffee creamer, mayonnaise, and chips. For each of these food items, find a comparable replacement. Pudding can become low-fat pudding; instead of coffee creamer use skim milk. Whatever it is, don't just completely take it out of your diet. Swap it with something you really like instead. Otherwise, your changes won't stick. This is not about denial; it's about making better choices.

Since fresh fruits and vegetables, especially raw, are healthy for you and add fiber to your diet, you do not need to write those down. However, if you are eating 10 oranges a day, then you might want to look up the calories in an orange (it's 60). If you put anything on the fruits or vegetables (like butter), write that down.

It's important that you write down the calorie amounts without judgment, because the more you think of yourself as wrong for the foods you eat, the less honest you will be. Try to be like a private detective looking over a crime scene. You are simply observing so that you can understand the situation better. This process is for your best interests and not to be seen as punishment. I know for some of my clients, it was a huge eye opener because, like many of us, they simply didn't know what was in the food they ate. Reading labels and becoming aware of calories and fat takes practice, but it's a habit I strongly recommend you develop—starting now.

If you are going to make this weight-loss process work long term, you have to find a way to make elements of it work automatically. For example, rather than trying to budget calories with each and every meal and snack, try to create new habits around eating so that you don't have to do a lot of thinking about it. One way is to make lower calorie choices in general. But that starts with knowing how many calories are in the foods you eat every day, so you can decide what's really important to you.

It's not just the big things that make the difference between being fat or thin. It's the little things you do every day that determine your size. Find a way to cut 500 easy calories out of your daily diet and you will lose one pound per week. It's not as hard as you think.

Eat Less Sugar

I had always heard that if you stop eating sugar, you stop craving it, but I really didn't believe it until I experienced it for myself.

After a lingering health issue, my doctor recommended I go on a special diet for a while that required me to cut out coffee and refined sugars in all their forms. I barely heard him say "no sugar" and focused on the "no coffee." I asked, "Are you insane? Do you realize how addicted to coffee I am? It's going to be awful!" He correctly predicted, "As addicted as you think you are to coffee, you are probably 10 times more addicted to sugar." Since I thought I didn't eat a lot of sugar, his prediction made no sense, but I decided to follow his advice and start the diet. He was so very right. Giving up coffee was nothing compared to how hard it was to give up sugar.

I discovered when I started *really* checking labels, sugars (sugar, sucrose, high-fructose corn syrup, evaporated cane juice, etc.) are in almost everything. Even things you might not expect, like bread and catsup. It took me a full week just to pull everything out of my diet with sugar in it. I had to replace my ice cream with frozen grapes, the sugar in my oatmeal with raisins, and my post-dinner dessert with sugar-free dried fruit. I learned that fruit smoothies with a little bit of Stevia are really good.

And I am not going to lie—it was tough. I had never been a big sugar eater, or so I thought, but my body was used to getting some every day, and that addiction was more than just psychological. This scared me because I really don't like the idea of being addicted to anything, particularly something that is in so many things we eat every day.

The diet lasted one month, and over that time a small miracle happened. After a couple of weeks, I realized I had stopped craving sugar. Once I stopped eating it, my body stopped expecting it, and the cravings went away. Then when I could eat it again, I found that everything with sugar just seemed too sweet and didn't really even taste good. Even the spiced Chai from the coffee shop that never seemed to have any sugar in it before suddenly tasted too sweet, and I didn't like it anymore. After that I decided to cut back on sugar permanently, and it has completely changed my diet for the better. I was eating healthy before, but now it's so much better, and I can really feel the difference in my body. My energy levels stay steadier throughout the day, which helps me eat less in general.

My suggestion is that you find ways to remove the bulk of the sugar from your diet. It could be difficult at first because we are so used to sweet comfort foods being a big part of our diets, but after a couple of weeks, you really won't even miss it. The rewards for changing your diet that way are tremendous and can really turn your life around for the better. I hope you will give it a try. The following meditation should help.

Meditation: Cutting Back Sugar

Allow yourself to relax and focus your attention inside. Go even deeper by using *the deepening process* from earlier in the book.

Picture yourself on a beautiful day. It's warm and clear outside, and your body feels so healthy and strong walking in this beautiful natural place. As you walk along the beach feeling so at peace and healthy, think about all the things you can eat, things your body likes, that make you feel healthier and stronger, and that keep your mind clear, for example healthy lean meats, fresh vegetables, and healthy grains. Notice how much better your body feels when you even think about those foods. Also notice how much lighter you feel with those foods in your mind. Life-affirming foods allow you to achieve your goal of being the healthiest version of yourself, and your body loves it when you feed it healthy food.

Because you like how you feel with healthy foods, you now find yourself drawn more and more to that way of eating. In fact, you would rather eat the healthiest foods possible all of the time in quantities that are good for you.

Now imagine some of the other foods you eat, particularly sugary foods. Notice how sluggish you feel when you think of those foods. In the past, you many have found them very appealing, but now you find they have no appeal at all. In fact, as you become aware of how they make you feel—tired, sluggish, less alive, fat, and unhealthy—you no longer want to put very much of them in your body at all. You find that instead of craving sweets that don't make you feel good, you now choose a piece of healthy fruit when you want something sweet. When you eat a piece of healthy fruit, you feel so strong, so alive and so good inside.

As you continue along your path on the beach on this beautiful day, you find that your craving for sweet foods diminishes more and more with each step you take. You know that you can have something sweet if you want but now you choose life-affirming foods that make you feel healthy and strong inside. Take a few more steps and feel any cravings you have for sugars leave your body. After a few more steps, see yourself automatically choosing healthy foods, knowing that each additional step brings you closer to the healthiest version of your body, and that feels so good inside. As you walk even further down the beach, know that you are moving toward health and away from your old habits and into the new healthy happy you inside.

Now that you are feeling healthier and stronger inside, open your eyes and immediately drink a nice cool refreshing glass of water to refresh yourself.

Summary

Being healthy is about being aware of what you are eating. Don't obsess and worry about the amount of calories in every little thing you put in your mouth like gum (10 calories). But just like you wouldn't want your young child to eat something without knowing what was in it, don't allow yourself to eat a type of food unless you have made sure you feel OK with the amount of calories and fat that's in it. You can still have the food item if you want, but bringing awareness to it empowers you and makes it about choosing rather than finding out later, for example, your favorite smoothie has 700 calories and 30 grams of fat in it. If that's the case, maybe you don't need it every day, or maybe you share it with a friend. But either way, it's about what's best for you. Love yourself enough to pay attention to what you put into your sacred self.

Lesson 8: Portion Sizes

Now that you have started the process of bringing awareness to the calories in the food you are eating and have begun swapping out some of your higher calorie items for lower ones, it's time to start looking at your portion size.

My sister-in-law is from the Philippines, and when she first got here she mentioned how surprised she was by how much food we eat. She referred to our portion sizes as "American sizes" since, even though the Philippines has some of the same chain restaurants as we have here, a "large" for them is usually equivalent to our "small." Americans comparably eat very large portions, and those sizes are growing bigger and bigger every year. At many fast food restaurants here, you can't even buy a small drink or fries unless you get a kids meal.

I think that's because we are so used to eating large portions, we have lost perspective on what a healthy portion looks like and how much we really should be eating. It may be part of our culture and is even seen as manly (e.g., Hungry Man dinners) to eat very large portions, but our bodies are paying the price. In general, almost everyone should be eating smaller portions, but that would mean adjusting both our bodies and our minds. Consider the actual amount of food our bodies actually need to feel full or satisfied, and this is where many diets fail.

The Real Reason Most Diets Fail

The problem with the typical weight-loss diet model is that when we go from eating 3,000+ calories a day down to the 1,200-1,500 calories most diets put you on, your body will have some trouble adjusting to that food amount, and because of such a dramatic change, you will feel hungry all the time, moody, and sometimes light-headed. This discomfort usually results in us tossing out our diet plans and going back to the old ways.

Your mind also needs time to adjust. When you look at a smaller portion of food on your plate, your mind sees it as an insufficient amount and starts thinking you are going to starve. It then dwells on what you can't have, and you become concerned about how miserable your body will feel if that's all you can eat. Usually that puts an end to your diet plans.

To lose weight and keep it off, you have to work in harmony with your body rather than against it by gradually dropping your portion sizes down so that your body can adjust to the feeling of being satisfied with smaller amounts, and your mind can look at your plate without thinking about starvation.

The Easiest Diet to Follow Ever Created

You began the first part of this process in the last exercise. Now it's time to start swapping out your high-calorie foods for some low-calorie options, and start cutting back on soda, juice and alcohol consumption if you haven't already. Again, don't take anything completely out or this won't work. It may take a few weeks to really make those adjustments, but you should begin to see some weight loss pretty quickly, particularly if you are able to nearly eliminate your soda.

After a few weeks of this, the next step is to take whatever you are currently eating and only consume only 80% of it. That should satisfy you without making you feel full. Though this seems so simple, it's actually not easy to do, so you have to be very meticulous about it. Here are a few pointers:

- Cut off 1/5 of your lunchtime sandwich (that's slightly less than 1/4).
- Either load up your plate with 20% less food or leave 20% on your plate (saving the leftovers for another meal).
- If you eat cereal, don't fill up the bowl or use all the milk you normally would.

- If you eat a candy bar, cut 20% off the end and give it to a friend.
- If you get a fancy coffee drink, either order a smaller size, or drink only 80% of it. The same is true for anything else you drink except water.

Eating 20% less of everything means, in some cases, not finishing all that's in the bag, but it's important that you learn to throw it away even if there is still some left. This is the first step in eating less food, and for a lot of my clients, this is the only thing they have to change to lose weight.

Initially you may find that you still feel hungry, but keep in mind, if you are overweight you have been eating more food than your body needed, and it has grown accustomed to that larger amount. It now needs time to get used to that smaller amount. Wait 20 minutes after your meal and, if you still feel hungry, allow yourself to have a little bit more or, even better, eat some plain healthy vegetables—plain meaning no butter or sauce other than low-cal dressing. By telling yourself you can have more in 20 minutes if you really need it, you keep yourself from experiencing that urgent feeling that the fear of a lack of food may cause. Most likely after you have had a glass of water at the end of your meal and allowed your food to settle, you will feel plenty full and will probably even forget that you wanted more. The best part is your body will have started the process of expecting less food, so you will get the "satisfied" signals sooner.

By making this change, you should really start to see some weight coming off, and this should continue for a while, longer if you get some exercise. However, after a few months you may begin to plateau and not see any weight loss for a couple of weeks. When this happens, it's time to cut 20% of your new lower amount out of your diet. It's been my experience working with clients that going below 1,500 calories for women or 1,800 calories for men is a really hard level to maintain, so I wouldn't recommend going that low. Check with your doctor to determine the lowest calorie levels that would be safe for you, however most people are eating way more than those amounts and have room to spare.

Since your weight gain is probably the result of gradually eating more and more food over time, you need to gradually step down from this overeating in order to make the new habits stick. In my experience, radical new diets have little staying power. Starving yourself will never work for very long; simply putting less on your plate will help you start feeling more comfortable with less.

One final reason cutting back slowly is best is because when we dramatically reduce the calories we eat, our body's metabolism naturally goes into "starvation mode," where it slows down (as it would during a famine in the old days), making it even harder to succeed in losing weight. A more gradual approach prevents this from happening.

The following meditation should help you cut back the 20%.

Meditation: 80% of Food

When you are ready, find a time you can relax and focus inside. Use the deepening process from earlier in the book to go even deeper.

As you allow yourself to relax and drift deeper, see yourself on a beautiful beach. It's a sunny day, and you can smell the ocean air, hear the waves crashing, and feel a gentle breeze on your face. See yourself with eyes closed, taking it all in. Now I want you to tap into the feeling of self-love and self-acceptance. Perhaps you can imagine a time when you felt loved and accepting of yourself and your body. Now allow yourself to feel an even greater sense of self-love as you open your heart to this feeling of self love more fully. Listen to the waves, and with each wave feel even more waves of self-love—love of your body, mind, and self.

Now focus on the feeling of loving your body and wanting to take care of its health. Become aware that your body needs certain amounts of food to be in its healthiest state. In the past you had been feeding it too much, sometimes unhealthy food, but now that you are more connected to how much you love yourself and your body, you want it to have what it needs to be healthy.

Imagine in front of you a dial that controls the amount of food you want to eat. See yourself turning down the dial and changing the overall amount to 80% of what you are eating now. Eating 80% is more than enough to keep your body healthy and nourished. Become aware of how much better and healthier your body feels inside when you feed it only 80% of what you had been eating. Also, notice how much stronger it is when it's not weighed down by too much food. Your body glows at that lower food amount, and you are more energetic with those smaller portions.

Now visualize yourself eating a healthy meal and only eating 80% of what you had been eating, yet feeling fulfilled at that amount. You know you can always have more if you want, but you feel so much better with less that it doesn't even feel comfortable anymore to eat what you had been eating. Also, see yourself eating more slowly and drinking more water than before, drinking a full glass of water at the end of every meal so that your body can get all the hydration it needs to process your food and turn it into usable energy.

You now feel so comfortable and so free with those smaller portions. You love yourself and your body enough to make those changes in a way that your body can easily accept. You know that keeping your body healthy and properly fed is the best way to feel loved and protected inside.

When you feel complete, open your eyes and feel yourself and your body adjusting to this new way of being.

Summary

Creating the habit of eating less food and getting used to smaller portions is one of the best and easiest ways to lose weight. By doing this you are working with your body rather than against it, and since the change is so gradual it shouldn't be too difficult or painful for the body. This may seem like a longer approach than more drastic and immediate calorie restriction, but consider this: for most people, that more extreme approach isn't something they are able to maintain, so even though they may lose more weight initially, they can't keep it up, and that's simply not a lifelong solution. Over the next few weeks, work on this gradual step down and watch your body start to change.

Lesson 9: The Roles We Give Food

Food has gotten a bad rap, and many of us who spent long periods of time on diets learned to both love and hate food because it also represents fat. But it's really not the food itself that is the enemy; it's the overinflated value we put on it, both as a culture and as individuals, that causes our problems with food. Food's real role should only be sustenance and refreshment and occasionally (in a healthy way) a way of connecting and bonding and sharing experiences (i.e., sitting around the dinner table with family and friends). But for most of us, food exceeded those few roles a long time ago as it started to become the center of our universe and for some people, an almost full-blown obsession.

We have made food very powerful by giving it so many roles in our lives, and that is really where the problem resides, not the food itself. Below, I've briefly outlined some of these alternate roles we give food, after which I discuss some of them in more detail.

What Food Has Become for Many of Us

Drug of choice. We use food as a way of managing feelings we don't want to feel. When we are dealing with strong and difficult emotions of us reach for food as a way of tuning out or calming feelings we may not be equipped to handle. Not only does this keep us from learning how to handle our feelings in a healthy way but it can have disastrous consequences on your health.

As celebration and connection with family. Birthday cake, holiday candy, Christmas cookies, wedding cake, graduation dinners—these are just some instances where food is used as a way of celebrating special moments with friends and family. There is nothing wrong with this, except when it results in us associating cake and other sweets with feelings of being happy, so much so that when we want to feel happy, we run to sweets, and that's when our relationship with sweets truly becomes out of balance.

Entertainment. Chips and dip with the big game, beer and the weekend barbeque—these are other opportunities in which we use a social event as an excuse to gorge ourselves with food and that is really unhealthy.

A buffer at social events: Eating gives us something to do during the inevitable awkward silence that comes before or after "So what do you do for a living?" And nobody, and I really mean nobody, wants to look silly or foolish in front of strangers. So we head over to the hors d'oeuvres bar and load up on some of the unhealthiest food available and end up eating huge amounts of it. The overeating usually happens because we are so nervous that we miss the "Stop, I'm full!" signals that our bodies are trying desperately to send us.

Food as love: We learn at an early age that certain foods are given out of love. Remember those Valentine's Day candy hearts? Grandma's special cookies she made for you to show she cared. They are all so effective at connecting the concepts of love and food for many of us, even the thought of chocolate chip cookies can brings up feelings of love. We'll delve deeper into this in the section on emotions and food, but for now it's important to be aware of the role we give food.

Distraction: Ever eat when you are bored? I do. One of my clients called it "foraging". For some, it's an automatic response when you find yourself with nothing to do, particularly in the mid afternoon.

Tool for beating self up: Of all the things food has become, this is truly the most destructive. When we make ourselves feel bad about eating food we set up a vicious cycle of eating, beating ourselves up for doing it and then running for food to soothe that hurt. The struggle and upset around food, overeating and binging is a bit like glue holding the habit of overeating in place and it has to stop if you want to keep the weight off for good.

A way of stuffing down your truth: This one is harder to explain, but most of us do it. What I call "stuffing your truth" is when you unconsciously suppress your inner needs to express yourself to the outside world. If you grew up in a family where expressing your feelings and opinions was not allowed, you may have created a habit of putting food in your mouth instead of speaking up for yourself and possibly facing punishment or ridicule. Often when overweight people really start standing up for and expressing themselves, their weight just melts away.

Now let's take a closer look at each of the above to gain a better understanding how and why we use food so destructively:

Food as Drug of Choice

Everyone learns different ways of handling difficult emotions. People who grew up in more functional families are taught to turn to positive coping mechanisms, like talking with others, journaling, or exercise. Others who did not learn healthy ways of handling emotions often turn to drugs, alcohol, or shopping; but almost everyone at some point turns to food.

Using food as my drug of choice to cope with an unhappy childhood was a major reason I was overweight. My home life was the source of much unhappiness in my early years and severe depression in my teen years. I have mentioned before that my father had a violent temper, and at a very young age I learned to greatly fear him. Even when he wasn't angry, he was very far from being loving or nurturing. Home for me was not a physically or emotionally safe place, and I often dreaded getting off the school bus at the end of the day to return to that hostile environment. Sometimes after checking in I would find some food, and then go hide so I could do my homework in relative safety.

In the days before Oprah and self-help books, I knew of no other way to manage my feelings than to eat, and though it didn't solve anything, it did make me feel better for a little while—at least long enough for me to calm down and get past the worst of my feelings. Food became my best friend and one of the few things I took real pleasure in. When I had food in my hand, I felt grounded and stable. When there wasn't food around, I felt anxious, as though I needed it's presence to survive. That may sound a bit like addiction, and in a sense, for me, it was.

In my young life there were few things I had any control over, but because it was impossible for my parents to watch my every action, food and eating seemed like something I could control, at least somewhat. And as a result, I gave food a more important role in my life than I should have. Though it did make me feel better for a short time, it also made me fat. And because I had food, I didn't learn other, more healthy ways of handling my emotions—ways that would have actually helped. The habit of reaching for food was the most ingrained of my negative habits, and consequently, the most difficult one for me to break. But I had to in order to not only lose weight, but also to learn to find solutions that actually helped me manage my emotions rather than make things harder in the long run.

Overcoming my dependence on food was a major challenge for me since it had occupied so many roles in my life. I had to untangle all those relationships I had created with food and find other ways of handling my life problems. I had to literally learn how to feed myself love in ways other than with food. I will get into those later, but for now I will just say that when I did stop using food to fill so many of my needs, I found it was actually very simple to lose weight. When food is no longer everything to you, it's easy to pass on the bread when you really don't need it and instead, focus your attention on the wonderful conversation at your table.

Food: A tool to beat yourself up with

Take an ordinary situation in life, like overeating at a party, and add emotions to it. Overeating at a party becomes, "I am such a huge pig. I can't believe I ate that whole piece of pie and those cookies and that soda. I am so fat and ugly I should be ashamed of myself. I have no self-control." Though that scenario may sound very close to the way you regularly speak to yourself, it's uncomfortable to hear. However, you should be aware that what really happened was you went to a party and ate more calories than you needed to satisfy your hunger. There is no meaning beyond the factual information until we assign it some, like making overeating at a party somehow be a sign that you are bad.

The worst part is that if we really listen to the words, we often realize they are actually things family members or bullies at school used to say to us. But now we have internalized that person in our life and become that bully. This is especially true if you grew up in a household where criticism and over concern about your appearance were the norm.

When we use food as a way of beating ourselves up, we begin to associate the act of eating with being criticized and feeling bad about ourselves. And what do we do when we feel bad about ourselves? We run to the cupboard for cookies so we can soothe the hurt we caused ourselves when we got upset about eating when we are overweight, which begins the cycle all over again.

Since this issue is so important, I have included a meditation to help you get past it. I recommend doing it a few times over the next several weeks and anytime when you feel yourself getting caught up in using food as a way to mistreat yourself.

Exercise: The Roles We Give Food

Over the next week I want you to think about all the different roles food plays in your life and the many ways you make food important beyond just sustenance. Write them down in your journal, seeing if you can come up with roles other than the ones discussed in this section.

After you have a complete list, I want you to think of other things you can do to fill the roles that food would normally fill for you. For the most significant recurring roles, try to find multiple solutions for how to handle it. Strategies like journaling, drinking a large glass of water, and taking a walk work for just about every role we give food; for others, you may need to be more creative.

Overcoming some of the roles will be harder than others, but the key here is to start noticing when you have assigned food a role, because simply noticing that behavior automatically causes you to begin to change it. For example, you won't be able to fool yourself anymore when you hit the snack table at a party. You'll know you aren't hungry, and you just wanted something to do with your hands. This is fine, but maybe a glass of water and some carrots will work just as well for that role as a brownie and a soda. The only difference is one behavior gets you closer to your goals and the other one, further away.

Here are some examples of the most common roles and suggestions for how to overcome them:

Drug of choice: Start by developing the habit of noticing when you are reaching for food when you are upset and start thinking of other things you can do: spending time with family, going for a walk, or reading a book are great temporary fixes.

A tool for beating yourself up: I will talk about this more in-depth in section about words, but for now your best strategy is to catch yourself doing it and decide to be kinder to yourself instead. You can choose to treat yourself with love and respect no matter what. Make that choice now and practice being more loving to *you.*

Celebration with family and friends: It's OK to enjoy a good meal, but try not to let it be the center of the activities. The best birthday party I went to as a child was one for a child with diabetes. When we got there, we were greeted with an assortment of outdoor toys—balls, Frisbees, squirt guns—lots of fun energetic things to do. There was food at the event, but it wasn't the centerpiece; the activities were, and that was so much more fun than eating a big piece of cake while sitting around in the living room. I suggest that you always plan on some kind of activity after every celebration meal, whether it's volleyball or football in the backyard or a nice walk at a local park. It helps to anchor the idea that celebration is not just about food it's about physical activity. Bringing sport to a family event is not only healthier; it's a great bonding tool.

Something to do at a social event: I got this idea from a friend of mine, who is a recovering alcoholic. It's a way to prevent someone from offering you a beverage when you first walk into an event: simply bring your own large coffee or bottle of water. That way you already have something to do with your hands, and you won't be tempted to grab food just to keep busy. Also, look for some kind of healthy vegetable you can nibble on, but on the off-chance there won't be any, just eat a big meal before you arrive so you'll be less tempted to eat anything at the event, because once you start, it can be hard to stop.

Food as love: The best way to break this one is to stop giving yourself food when you want love. More on this later, but for now if you want to nourish yourself take a nice bubble bath or plan some time off. This is a habit that is best broken by simply stopping the behavior cold. Also, you'll need to ask your loved ones not to give you candy and sweets as gifts. I have told all my boyfriends, and now my husband, that I love all kinds of gifts, but please no candy, because it doesn't help me achieve my highest goals. Most people will respect your wishes if you tell them. Be creative. It's fun to give yourself love in ways that won't make you unhealthy.

Distraction: Ah, eating because you are bored. Catching yourself doing this is the best trigger for realizing you need something else to do. If I find myself foraging in the cupboards for food, I know I need more stimulation in my life. Perhaps it's time to crack open a good book, start a creative project, or simply go for a walk, whatever will get you out and feeling interested in life again.

Stuffing your creative ideas or feelings: You will never be truly happy in life if you consistently stuff your feelings, your creative ideas, or needs with food rather than expressing them. There is simply no way around that. You have so many special gifts to share with the world, and by keeping your gifts to yourself you are depriving the world of your special light. Everyone has the right to reach their highest potential, and that needs to start by you doing that for you.

If you know this is one of your big problems, and for some reason you don't feel safe expressing yourself, it might be a good idea to connect with a counselor who can help you get past this habit and figure out why you aren't feeling free to be your true self. The easiest and safest way to start the process of expressing yourself is by creating a journal or sketchbook where you can put down your ideas and feelings.

Meditation: Severing Your Feelings about Food

Allow yourself to comfortably relax and focus inward. Now relax even deeper using *the deepening process* from earlier in this book and see yourself entering a beautiful place inside—it's your place of contemplation, where you go to make decisions and find resolution. Imagine it as a room with a giant table full of your favorite foods. Now, as you focus just on the food, notice if there are any feelings associated with specific foods or types of foods. If there isn't, just notice your feelings about foods in general.

See those feelings and emotions as strings attached to the food, causing the food to be more important to you in your life than it really is. Then think about the roles you have assigned those foods. As you relax a bit deeper, you start to see that the food itself can never serve a role in your life other than satisfying hunger as you imagine all those other roles being handled in different and healthier ways.

Now that you have decided to use food for sustenance only, you are able to get rid of the emotional strings attached to the food. Imagine yourself now cutting all those emotional strings attached to the food, detaching yourself from all the emotions about the food, so that when you look at a particular food item you are able to see it for what it is rather than the emotions surrounding it. Take special note of any feelings of fear, urgency, or anxiety attached to the food, and sever those ties. Keep severing the ties until you are able to look at the table piled high with your favorite foods and feel neutral—so neutral that you can simply take it or leave it depending on whether you are hungry or not.

Now that you are feeling more neutral about food, see yourself enjoying healthy versions of what you really like: low-fat ice cream, low-fat dressings in much smaller portions. Also, visualize yourself adding lots of fresh fruits and vegetables to your favorites, especially things you have never tried before as you explore many of the flavorful healthy vegetables available. Because you are more neutral about food, you are able to make healthier and more life-affirming choices. You can still have everything you like, but you see yourself now preferring foods that are more in line with your goals. Feel yourself becoming more and more content with healthier food choices.

When you feel good about the food choices on your table, open your eyes to this new way of feeling about food and resolve to add into your diet some of your new, healthier choices.

Summary

The easiest way to end a behavior is to first notice yourself doing it. As I mentioned before, awareness is the key to change, and it starts when you pay attention to all the roles you give food and how you make it too important in your life. Food is just sustenance; and if you want to have a healthier, more balanced relationship with it begin by reminding yourself of that.

Lesson 10: Food—Lack and Control

In the last section I talked about how we make food too important by giving it multiple roles in our lives and using it as tool for making ourselves feel bad. The biggest way we create upset and make food extremely important is by trying it exercise "self-control," which in my opinion is the number one reason we fail in our weight-loss efforts. Control, when it comes to food, is a losing battle. You aren't overweight because you lack control, but because something else is out of balance in your life. Let me explain.

When you were a child, did you ever have one of those Chinese finger puzzles? This was a paper tube that you put one finger from each hand into and then tried to pull them out. The more you pulled outward, the more the tube tightened, making it impossible to get your fingers out because you were pulling against yourself. The trick was to push both fingers toward the middle of the tube, and then you were free to go. It's the same way for your weight: you will not win this game by fighting yourself or fighting for control.

Fighting for control, self-control, creates tension and upset which eventually causes you to eat more. We as human beings hate control, and it's in our nature to push back against it when it comes up. But you have to learn to work with yourself by understanding and respecting all parts of you, even the part that wants a cookie—you don't have to give it one, but you do have to listen. Remember, unless you have physical hunger, you never *need* food for anything; it's always just a crutch.

Contrary to popular belief, fat people do not lack self–control. In fact in some cases they exert more control over themselves than most people. After all, they normally don't turn around and hit the person who asks them, "Do you really need another cookie?" though I am very sure they often want to. In reality, overweight people try to control every bite they put in their mouth. They usually lose that battle, but most of the time they put a lot of thought and effort into it.

Thin people, by contrast, do not try to control what they eat as much as they just make more life-affirming choices. This can be easier for a thin person because they do not feel the desperation of being overweight that causes them to feel bad about themselves and pushed to control what they eat. Self-control will never make you stay thin for very long, and if it does, it certainly won't make you happy—just ask any young woman with anorexia or bulimia. However, giving yourself what you really need inside and engaging all parts of your personality in the weight-loss process will make you happy.

One of the reasons self-control doesn't work is because controlling what you eat involves focusing on what you can't have, what's been taken away, and staying away from the "bad" or "forbidden" food rather than learning to be satisfied with healthier portions of healthier foods. When you say "no" to what you desire, you are immediately creating resistance in yourself against the part that wants it, and that tug of war, or Chinese finger puzzle, as many of you have experienced, is a losing battle of wills. Becoming satisfied with more life-affirming choices and the goal you are trying to reach is what will bring you long-term success, not control.

"Lack" and Controlled Substances

What happens when you tell a three year old "no" when he or she asks for a candy bar in the store? Does the young child listen quietly to your explanation that it's not healthy, accept what you say as gospel, and then calmly tell you, "That makes sense. You are right; candy isn't good for me. I don't want it anymore. Thanks for letting me know"? Absolutely not! The child will usually complain loudly, cry, or scream and sometimes even try to negotiate, "Pa-leeese mommy! But I really *really* want it. I'll be really good." Whether or not the child really does want it, the reason it really really "needs" it is because you have unwittingly done what marketing firms have been doing since advertising began: by saying "no," you made that food item very special, more special than it was before your child asked for it. You have made it scarce, the most coveted of all marketing ploys. In other words, denying the candy creates a sense of *lack* around it, thus making the food item, in a sense, a controlled substance. It's similar to when something is in short supply or is only available for a short time, like Christmas cookies and eggnog—it suddenly has more perceived value.

We see this all the time in toy marketing. When I was young, the big toy every child wanted was the Cabbage Patch Kids. They were just ordinary dolls that were kind of cute and came with a birth certificate and unique name, but otherwise they were nothing special. But when every child started asking for them when the stores only had a "limited supply," the price shot way up, and people would do anything to get one. They suddenly became much more valuable than they would have been if there were plenty and people weren't waiting in line for hours at stores so they could buy one.

Similarly, foods like holiday cookies, which are only available at certain times of year, are considered "special" and are specifically tied to celebration, thus putting you in the position of saying "no" to both *controlled* and *special.*

Even worse, the most controlled and special foods generally fall into one certain category—sweet. We almost never control the amounts of a healthy food a child might want, giving it no value in a child's mind even if it's something it likes. One client told me her dad hated Brussels sprouts, so her mom never made them unless he was out of town, which was rare. As a result, that food became special, and it's still one of her favorites. This is an unusual example of a healthy food becoming special, but her story illustrates that actions taken around the food, and not the particular food itself, can make that food item more desired.

So now, in the mind of the child who's begging for candy this entire category of food has become extremely valuable because 1) by deciding when they can have it, we have made it a controlled substance (remember, it's human nature to push back against control); 2)and by controlling the item, particularly if the child has actually seen it, we have created a shortage or lack in its world; and 3) this serves to reinforce the idea of certain foods being "special" by calling them special and only serving them on "special" occasions.

So what does this have to do with me? I'm not a child anymore. Well, you are and you aren't. Your internally programmed ideas about how important food is, and your emotional attachments to specific foods, were created at a very young age and are still running the show. So now as an adult, you want to lose some weight and decide to go on a diet, which involves controlling your food portions, saying "no" to certain foods, and giving up things that are "special." However, the part of you that is still a child, holds on to ideas about how valuable food is, and doesn't like losing control. This part of you thinks certain foods are so special that you can't possibly live without them. Therefore the controls you place on your life as an adult feel a lot like the ones you hated as a child.

Instead of protesting against mom when you wanted candy, you are protesting against yourself; only now you have the power to win since you are physically capable of going to the store on your own and buying every candy bar, quart of ice cream, or chocolate chip cookie they sell. You may be able to fight and resist it for a while, sometimes even long enough to lose some weight, but ultimately the inner three year old will start whining again, and you will start craving all the foods you denied yourself. Eventually this will cause you to go off your diet and gain all the weight back, sometimes more.

How Do You Devalue Food?

The way to make something have less value to you is to reverse the "lack" by allowing yourself complete access to it. That means you need to take food off the "controlled substance list" and experience the freedom of eating what you want, whenever you want—with some rules, of course.

But, but, I can't do that!

Right now you may be thinking, "If I let myself eat whatever I want, I will go crazy and never stop eating." And don't be surprised if you do, in fact, eat a bit more for a few days, or even a week, while you adjust to this new way of being. But after a short time of letting yourself have what you want, the sense that food is special and controlled starts to diminish, and the food stops feeling so exciting, leaving you free to make healthier choices. This will happen once you start to notice, for example, that your body feels better when you eat carrots rather than cookies. Another reason this idea sounds crazy is that it runs completely against the advice about dieting and eating most of you have been given your entire life. But I promise you if you take on this challange, you will stop the push-pull relationship you have with food and be able to release your urgent feelings about having it.

But that doesn't make sense!

If diamonds were plentiful and, as a result, worth $3 rather than $3,000, would we still give them as a gift to show how valuable someone is to us? Probably not, but does that change the diamond any? No. Only the perceived value goes down. If cake, cookies, ice cream, were everywhere, and we could have them anytime we wanted, would they still be as special to us? Certainly we would still enjoy them, but they wouldn't be as special because of the tug of war game we play with food, —*can't have, bad for you, you are bad for eating it,*—would no longer be there for our emotions to get caught up in. Food is just sustenance, and that's all we should want it to be.

I encourage you to give this a try using the rules I have laid out below. If it doesn't work for you, it doesn't. However, consider that years of denial and struggle probably haven't worked either, and this change, as radical as it may sound, could change your life for the better.

Guidelines for Eating Whatever You Want
Don't do anything else while eating. That means no TV, talking on the phone, reading, or surfing the Internet. When

you eat, just eat and be fully present in this activity. You also want to practice eating consciously by eating more slowly. Take the time to notice the texture and flavors of the foods you are eating, the way they feel in your mouth. Notice how the meal smells, what the colors look like on your plate, and how your body feels while you are eating it. Taking the time to observe these things will automatically slow down your eating, and it will also help you feel more satisfied by your meal.

In addition, focusing on your eating and doing it more slowly helps you become more aware of your body's internal signals that tell you that you have eaten enough, signals you miss when you are distracted by entertainment. Most people go from full to stuffed very quickly because they were eating so fast they missed the first signal.

Buy small-sized "fun foods." When it comes to "fun foods" that have no real nutritional value, like chips, candy bars, or cookies, start with the smallest package available. For candy bars, that's the "fun" or "mini" size; for chips it's the kid-size packages. We are so programmed to feel

> *A word on chips*: Chemists and food scientists have figured out how to mix artificial flavors that you would never find in any kitchen that are so appealing to your taste buds you really can't eat just one.

that we are finished when we reach the end of the package, that often we feel done after finishing even the small packages. You can always go back and have more, but start with one or two very small portions and see if you want more later. Again, especially with "fun foods," it's very important that you eat them while not doing anything else.

Soda and juice are considered "fun foods." Sodas, energy drinks, and other sugary beverages, including juice (yes, even if it's 100% juice), have become what water should be: refreshment and hydration. The only hydration your body really needs is water. Drinks like soda and juice are really desserts and should be treated as thus.

Since soda with caffeine is addicting, I would highly recommend working on greatly reducing the amount you drink. In the case of juice, even though it may have some vitamins, it's basically sugar, and your body responds to it that way. An orange is a healthy food full of vitamins minerals and fiber; orange juice is dessert.

This Is an Important Process

I can tell you personally that this was the single most important change I made, and it is the reason I was able to lose the weight. I knew that saying "no" was only creating obsession, so I figured if I tried this approach and failed, it wouldn't be any different than saying "no" and inevitably failing at that. Part of my challenge, as I already explained, was the upset I created around food in general and the feelings of urgency for something I couldn't have. The other part was the obsession I had with sweet foods, as those were the foods I most denied myself, thus making them more important to me.

For example, I used to have a thing for candy bars, and I never "let" myself have one. This always generated an internal battle that usually ended with me going to the vending machine and getting one, then another, plus a bag of chips, all the while feeling very bad about eating like that, but unable to stop. When I decided to stop the fight and try my new approach, I bought two bags of assorted fun-sized candy and filled an entire desk drawer with them. The first day I probably ate ten, the next six or so, and it went down from there. Since I could have them whenever I wanted, it wasn't so special. After a while, a week would go by before I realized I hadn't eaten any. It just wasn't as much fun anymore if I could do it whenever I wanted. A candy bar you can have whenever you want doesn't taste as good to the inner saboteur as the one it forces you to eat in a sneaky way—more on that later.

Exceptions to the "eat whatever you want" rule: There are some people for whom this plan will not work. Certain people, due to a physical abnormality, are unable to receive any messages that they have eaten enough. Those people would never stop eating if they didn't place some kind of limit on the amount they ate.

Also, there are other people who report that they have particularly strong cravings for foods they are actually allergic to. I know for myself, being allergic to dairy, that if I have even a little cream or cheese, I find my cravings for it greatly increasing to a level that is hard to manage, so I just avoid it altogether and eat anything else I might want.

People with blood sugar imbalances of any kind may have very specific dietary restrictions that need to be adhered to in order to maintain optimal health regardless of any cravings they might have. In those cases, or if a doctor has put you on a specific diet for medical reasons, this process would not be for you. However, those cases are rare, and for most this should work.

If, after a couple of weeks, you haven't noticed any slowdown in the amount of food you are eating, then maybe this approach isn't for you. In that case, do use the other tools in the book to help you achieve your goals.

Can't stop foods: There is another exception to the "eat whatever you want rule." For almost everyone, there are a few foods that for various reasons once we start eating them, it's almost impossible to stop. These foods are not the same for everyone, or else I would list them here, but I suspect you can already think of at least one. For me it's cookies and a certain kind of really salty potato chip. Even now I still find it really hard to pull myself away from those foods once I start. I can stop eating almost anything else, but those two always get me.

My recommendation for those foods is to not even have them in the house. If you want them bad enough that you are willing to make a trip to the store, then let yourself have some, but don't make it too easy. And if you do decide to have some, buy the smallest package possible, like a snack pack. I never tell myself "no" to any food, because I don't want to create that tension, which ultimately leads to eating a lot of the food I am resisting. Although I don't keep those chips or cookies in the cupboard, I still have them sometimes. As I don't like the feeling that I can't stop eating something, I find it's best not to even start.

Exercise: Handling "Can't Stop" Foods

Think about the foods you know are almost impossible for you to stop eating. Then figure out something to replace that food with that's not so addictive to you but still has some of the same qualities of your "can't stop" food. For instance, I replace cookies with frozen grapes, which are crunchy and sweet like cookies, but don't make me feel like I can't stop eating them. I also replaced my salty chips with some low-fat microwave popcorn. It's crunchy-salty too, but I can definitely put the bag down after a short while.

My clients often tell me ice cream is their problem food. If that's the case, I would recommend switching to popsicles to see if that satisfies you. If that doesn't work, try Jell-O or pudding snacks. Others have difficulty with a particular kind of candy. If that's your problem treat, figure out what it is about that particular candy you really like and try to find a non-addictive replacement. This might take a bit of trial and error on your part, but eventually you can find a way to replace all those "can't stop" foods with things you can stop, but that also satisfy you.

Just as if you knew you were allergic to something, you wouldn't eat it, try thinking of these foods in that way, and it will make it easier to let them go.

Meditation: Food Is Plentiful—No Need to Feel Lack

This meditation will help you get in touch with the feeling that food is plentiful so you can take it or leave it, and you may as well just leave it. Do this meditation several times this week and anytime you start to feel any urgency with food. This meditation will help you feel on a core level that food will always be there, so there is no need to ever binge.

Sit and relax quietly and focus your attention on your breath. Notice the ebb and flow of each breath and allow your inhalation to bring in peace, relaxation and comfort while you allow each exhalation to help you relax more deeply inside. Now begin to find that place of inner nothingness using *the deepening process* from earlier in the book to more fully relax into it.

When you are ready, imagine yourself in a giant banquet hall full of large tables. See all your favorite foods piled high everywhere. On other tables, also see many different types of food, some very healthy, some not so healthy. Notice the abundance of food—there is plenty and you can have as much as you want because it will never run out.

As you allow yourself to relax a little deeper, you begin to realize that because there is so much food around you and so much abundance, no single food has more value than any other. Since that is the case, you may as well choose more of the foods that you like that also allow you to reach your goal of creating optimal health for yourself as quickly as possible.

Now see yourself choosing smaller portions of the more fatty, less healthy foods—yet not denying yourself anything—and choosing larger portions of the fruits, vegetables and lean meats. Feel that both those food choices are equal so you may as well have more of the foods that help you achieve your goals. Fill up on very small amounts of anything you like, knowing you can always have more, so there is no reason to stuff yourself now. See yourself eating more slowly and really savoring every bite, and, as you do so, find that you are paying more attention to your body and letting it tell you when it's full, all the while knowing that you can have more at any time, however you prefer to eat lighter since it makes you feel better.

When you feel satisfied and complete, open your eyes and begin your day.

Summary

There are no "bad" foods, only life-affirming and non-life–affirming ones. And unless you have a medical condition, like diabetes or food allergies, or your doctor says otherwise, it is ok to have a little candy bar once in a while.

It's not a bad thing, and you aren't bad for wanting it. An important part of this process is to separate out emotions from the food itself and see it simply as food rather than giving emotionally loaded traits like good or bad.

Again, to remove the specialness or value you have placed on certain food items, you must allow yourself to eat whatever you want. Don't be too surprised if you eat more than normal for a few days, though you may not. Your mind is just re-adjusting to the fact that you are no longer pulling on the rope in your tug of war game. Much like ending an argument by saying "You are right," and they turn and say "Are you serious?" like they're testing you as well. But if you hang in there and allow yourself to really feel that food is plentiful, it will become less special.

Lesson 11: Emotions and Eating

Actual physical hunger, for many people is really only a small part of their desire to eat. Often we eat at certain times and certain amounts not from hunger, but from habit. Other times we eat as a result of our emotional state, and that is when we develop a problem.

When someone does not learn healthy ways of handling their emotions, they often turn to some unhealthy ones. For a lot of people, that is where emotional eating truly begins. Emotional eating is not about being hungry, but rather using food as a way of feeling better and it causes you to develop a very unbalanced relationship with food. And for many people I work with, this is the core reason why they are overweight and the source of much unhappiness in their lives.

What makes this issue especially difficult is that to some extent almost all eating is emotional. Even your basic family meal is an important time, it feels good to connect with loved ones and bond while doing something we have to do anyway—eat. That feeling is what we really seek, not the food. However, through years of bonding over food, we have conditioned ourselves to associate feelings of love, connection, and companionship with food. And then, when we want to feel those emotions again, instead of calling a friend, we often seek the food. This is especially true during times of upset in our lives when things feel out of control. Eating something can distract you long enough to be able to calm down a bit and to gain control of your emotions. The worst part of this cycle is that to some extent, it works—at least temporarily.

Unfortunately, eating to help you change or suppress your feelings keeps you from getting real help to solve your challenges. People who use food as a way of handling some of life's toughest emotional challenges miss the chance to learn the beneficial skill of handling their emotions in a healthy way. It's like taking an aspirin for a broken arm: it might take the pain away for a while, but it won't heal the injury. Similarly, there are many healthy long-term solutions to handling life's challenges, and trust me on this one, eating has never solved any problem—ever.

For me this was a very big problem. As I explained earlier, like many people, I grew up in a dysfunctional family and I had never been taught a healthy way of handling my feelings so when I got upset, I did what I had seen my mom do many times, I ran for food, and this became a near lifelong habit. I reached for food when I was angry, upset, and lonely. Food became my counselor and best friend, and I ate a lot of it. Whenever I would have a strong emotion, even if I had just eaten, I would suddenly become very hungry and devour something often without really tasting it.

Like most people, upsets were bad, but feelings of boredom were my real enemy, since it drove me to eat more than anything else. I grew up in rural Arkansas, in an area with no local libraries, playgrounds, or big towns nearby. Often, especially during the summer I would find myself with nothing, not even TV to occupy my very active mind. So I turned to food as something to do. And thus the habit of eating for entertainment developed. Even when I became an adult and could easily find other interesting things to do, that habit was so ingrained and automatic, eating was always the first thing I did when I was bored.

Food never solved any of my problems and never entertained me for more than a few minutes. The one and only thing it ever did was make me fat. In order to lose weight, I had to dismantle my previous habits and learn ways of managing my emotions that would actually resolve my issues and allow me to have the body and life I wanted.

For many of my clients, even just talking about emotional eating brings up emotions. People describe feeling very out of control with food, almost as though it has taken over their lives. I often hear about the embarrassment of being at a social event, eating nonstop, and thinking people are talking about them behind their backs, all the while they are feeling completely powerless to control their behavior. Often eating is the only tool that people have ever learned to handle challenging emotional situations.

One of the hardest things you will have to do to in order to create the body you want is to break the habit of emotional eating. But it is imperative that you break yourself of this habit as part of your journey. You can do this, and in the next few sections I will show you how.

Emotional Eating from Deeper Emotions

Emotional eating is unconscious, meaning you aren't thinking about it; you are just reaching and eating. Sometimes whatever feelings you are experiencing in the moment, like boredom or loneliness, is driving your emotional eating. Other times it can be specific life situations, like an unsatisfying romantic relationship or being unhappy at your job. But the most difficult triggers to deal with are the emotions that come from deeper unhealed wounds of the past, such as those from an abusive childhood or spending your entire life suppressing your true self. For example in the case of an artist who denied that part of him- or herself to make more money working in an unfulfilling corporate job.

Whatever place these emotions come from, it's tempting to continue the habit of stuffing away your unhappiness with food while refusing to face some unpleasant realities in your life. However facing them will free you from more than just the fat. When you no longer stuff those feelings away with food, you will be able to make important life changes, which could lead to true happiness.

I worked with a woman who was the mother of two young children. She had recently discovered her husband was cheating on her, but for many reasons she was not ready to confront him, including the possible destruction of her family. So instead of handling her feelings, she ate and ate, eventually packing on an additional 20 pounds to her already overweight body. Since her husband had told her many times that her weight made him feel less attracted to her, this devastated her already damaged self-esteem.

With help, she was able to acknowledge how she felt, even though she still wasn't ready to kick her husband to the curb. She did, however, start taking steps to protect herself, including looking for a job, figuring out a childcare arrangement, and working with a good family therapist to help her decide if her relationship could be saved. This made her feel less like a victim and more like a woman taking charge of her life, - truly powerful place to be. As she made these changes she started to lose the weight, but more importantly, she began rediscovering her feelings of self worth and self respect. All those positive changes started with bravery and being able to examine and confront issues in her life.

In the case of intense feelings of pain from past hurts or abuse in any form, seeking the help of a therapist is good way to begin to free the part of you that is trapped in that trauma and still reliving it. This is the part you may be trying to silence with food because you don't know any other way of handling those feelings. However, food won't help you heal past trauma or intense feelings of pain; but facing those feelings and getting help will. I always recommend the services of a good therapist since many of my very overweight clients were victims of sexual violation earlier in their lives. A therapist can really help you heal those wounds.

Emotions Are Your Friend—Spend Time with Them

Just like the best friend in your life who calls to tell you all about her problems, not to have you solve them, but just to be heard, sometimes the way to work through your emotions is just to be there for yourself while feeling them in a loving way. Try sitting in a hot bubble bath while you cry your eyes out over something that made you sad, talking your upsets out with your journal, or just sitting quietly and allowing those feelings to just be there without judgment and remind yourself "This too shall pass." My personal favorite way of handling anger is going for a run while thinking about how angry I am at that person, really helps me feel better. Emotions are not something to suppress or be afraid of, they are just energy, and the more you allow those feelings to be experienced and move through you, the less likely you will feel the need to use food as a way of managing them.

Anger

When it comes to anger in particular, I hear a real reluctance from people to feel it, and I can understand those feelings very well. With anger there is often the fear that if we really look at why we are angry, we might lose control or never stop feeling angry. If you have buried anger about the past, taking a look at those feelings and allowing yourself to process them can be upsetting take and long time. It can feel like clearing trash out of a closet that is five miles long. But in order for you to truly feel free to be yourself, you need to be able to look at those feelings, acknowledge them, and allow yourself to really get mad about what happened. Again, it would also be helpful to seek counseling to work through those feelings.

Think of pent up anger as stuck energy holding space in your mind as well as in your body. If you get that energy moving, you will not only release that anger, but you will have access to a great pool of energy you can use for other things.

Your emotions can't hurt you; they are not bad, nor are you wrong for having them. On the contrary, anger in particular is often your first clue that something is not right in your life, and it can be the greatest catalyst for change. Have you ever gotten really mad about something and then decided that drastic life changes were necessary? MADD (Mothers against Drunk Driving) was started by a woman who lost her son to someone who was driving under the influence. Similarly, many of the great stories of triumph were, in fact, the result of a defeat that created such a huge emotional upset that their life had to take a new direction.

Tools for Managing Anger

Just as with any emotion that causes you to eat, you need to create a plan for managing feelings of anger in a healthy way. And since anger is usually accompanied by a need to act out physically in some way, I recommend a physical activity to help you process those feelings.

Do intense physical activities like running, boxing, or a hard workout. While you work out, really feel your anger and allow yourself to get mad, and keeping up the intensity until those feelings begin to subside. Do this type of workout as often as you need to, it's a very therapeutic process that helps you release that pent up energy from your muscles and tissues, causing you to lose weight. Doing this was a key part in helping me get past my anger toward my dad so we could have a relationship again. I still do this to handle everyday angers and upsets. Trust me both your body and your mind will greatly benefit from the exercise.

Write out exactly how you feel. Write as much as possible as fast as possible so that your feelings just pour through your fingers onto the page. If doing this makes you feel even angrier, do some kind of physical exercise, but only after you have hand-written everything you can on paper. Make sure you write it by hand rather than typing it on your laptop. The physical act of writing moves that stuck energy in a way that typing does not.

Beat the stuffing out of one of your pillows. Think about what you are angry at and slam your fists into a pillow. If you feel the urge, yell and scream into it as well (quietly though so the neighbors don't call the cops). Trust me the pillow will survive.

Emotional clearing work. My hypnotherapist Michele Meiche created a great process on CD to help you neutralize the charge on your emotions. It's called the 5-step emotional clearing process. For more information visit her website at:

www.selfinlight.com

Also, on her website is another process I highly recommend for releasing emotional charge and getting to the heart of the matter.

http://www.soulinsights4spiritledliving.com/2011/10/projection-perception.html

Stop Emotional Eating

To put a stop to emotional eating, you need to develop four skills and habits:

1) **The ability to distinguish emotional hunger from physical hunger**. This takes practice, and I will show you how.
2) **The ability to observe your emotional states** while you eat, without judgment, so that you can catch yourself in the act.
3) **The ability to listen to your emotions** and what they are trying to tell you regarding your deeper unmet needs (hint: it's never about food).
4) **A plan** for other ways you can handle those feelings without needing to run to the kitchen cabinet for a food sedative.

Physical vs. Emotional Hunger

It's important for you to practice the skill of distinguishing between being physically hungry and emotional hunger. The differences can be very subtle, but those feelings are actually quite different, and with time, practice, and observation you can learn to feel the difference.

Unless you have a blood sugar imbalance, actual physical hunger is a more subtle physical sensation, sometimes a rumble in the stomach that builds and grows, becoming more intense as time goes on. Emotional hunger has a more compelling feeling to it, like "Gimmie that now or someone will die," it may feel as though the food has power over you. Also with emotional eating, you are drawn to very specific foods, like sweets or chips: "I am dying for French fries right now," or "I really really want mint chocolate chip ice cream." That feeling can be physical as well if your body is lacking certain nutrients, however if you've eaten recently and you're still craving "comfort food" that's a clue it might be emotional. Physical hunger is generally less specific, more like, "I really want lunch." Although you may prefer one thing over another on a particular day, like a turkey rather than a tuna sandwich, you are fine with either one.

When I first started working on this, I found it helpful to just close my eyes and ask myself, "Am I really hungry or am I just trying not to feel something?" (like boredom or loneliness). Initially when I did this, I would hear only silence in response to my question, but after a few weeks I started to hear myself answer. And if I was physically hungry, I would eat, often something healthier than what I initially wanted; if it was emotions, I would find other way of handling it that didn't have anything to do with food. In either case, it was about listening to my intuition and my needs and that was most important.

If distinguishing between physical and emotional hunger is a challenge for you, the following meditation should help you clarity your needs.

Meditation: Noticing Hunger

Allow yourself to relax and focus your attention on the inside using *"the deepening process"* from earlier in the book. Take a few deep breaths, following your breath inward as you relax even more deeply inside.

Now I want you to think of a time recently when you were hungry and wanted to eat your regular meal, a time when you were certain your hunger was physical. Perhaps it was your lunch time, and you were ready to eat. Get in touch with that feeling of being ready to eat. Notice how that feeling may have started earlier and continued to build as your lunch time got closer. As you tap into that feeling, I want you to take a mental picture that situation and of that feeling of physical hunger. Infuse that picture with all the feelings you were experiencing at the time notice what your body was experiencing, how your stomach felt. Set that picture and that feeling aside for the moment.

Now I want you to think about a time when you ate in response to a strong emotion or in response to being bored. Notice if your feelings of emotional hunger started and grew quickly and whether there was a particular type of food that you craved, for example something sweet or crunchy. Also notice if feeling was a bit more urgent and compelling. Recall whether you had taken a moment to think about the food you were reaching for or if it seemed to appear in your hands without much thought. As you tap into that scenario, take a mental picture of yourself in that scenario and infuse that picture with all the feelings you were experiencing at the time.

Now bring back the other picture of being physically hungry. See those pictures side by side and notice how those situations feel very different. Note any differences in the situations, like the cravings you may have had or how you felt afterward. Spend a few minutes becoming aware of what those two situations felt like.

Now that you really see these differences, it will be very easy for you to know when you are eating because of your emotions or because you are genuinely hungry.

When you feel very comfortable with your ability to tell the difference, open your eyes.

Observing Your Emotional State without Judgment

The first and probably most important requirement for looking at your different emotional states, particularly the ones you're trying to avoid by eating food, is courage. Emotions cannot harm you, but dealing with feelings of being hurt or sadness can be difficult if you have never learned any other way of coping with them rather than eating. After you learn to face your emotions and understand them, you'll grow more comfortable with allowing yourself to feel them, you may wonder why you were trying to stuff the emotions away with food.

Sometimes we're sad for no reason at all, but we shouldn't get upset with ourselves for feeling this way. Instead we should let those feelings be there without judgment and work through them without using food. When deny your emotions, it will become much harder to identify emotional eating and to shift to eating only when you are hungry.

Identifying Unmet Emotional Needs

Your emotions are powerful tools that can give you access to much more information than you realize, and you would be very wise to listen to them as much as you can. Your emotions are your inner-self asking for attention or letting you know something is wrong. Just as a child cries loudly when it needs something, your emotions are letting you know when you need something. Often when there is something inside you that is trying to be expressed, or an inner-nudging that something is wrong, it can feel like you are hungry all the time, and no amount of food will make that feeling go away.

For example, boredom is your minds way of saying *I need* something to stimulate me. Sadness or depression could be telling you something in your life is not working as it should be, like your relationship or your job. All of those things are valid issues and they cannot be resolved by eating.

Creating a Plan to Handle Your Emotions

You will need a plan to handle those emotions in a more healthy way, but since you can't resolve any challenge unless you fully understand it. You first need to tap into which emotions are driving your eating so that you can create new ways of handling them, a way that actually solves your problems rather than stuffing them away with food. There are ways of getting your real underlying emotional needs met that won't interfere with your need to create a lifetime of optimal health. The following assignment will help you 1) develop the habit of catching yourself when you emotionally eat; 2) become aware of which emotions are driving you to eat and your deeper emotional needs; and 3) develop a plan to create a more healthy way of being.

Exercise, Part 1: Understanding Your Emotional Eating

Take a small notebook that you can carry with you all day. Make a note every time you put something in your mouth.

Then check in with your emotions and ask yourself, "How am I feeling now?" Write down your feelings next to the food item.

If you have trouble identifying how you are feeling, try asking yourself, "What am I trying not to feel by eating?"

Some things will be neutral, especially meals like breakfast where we may eat the same thing every day. But if you normally have eggs and one morning decide to make pancakes, figure out which emotions may be driving that eating.

The next part is once you have identified which feelings are driving you to eat ask yourself, "What is it that I really need?" and write that down.

Your notebook page might look like this:

> Monday
> Breakfast — oatmeal, neutral
> Mid-morning — protein bar, bored. Real need: something to do.
> Lunch — sandwich & chips, neutral
> Post-lunch — donut, sad. Real need: companionship
> Mid-afternoon snack — chips, bored. Real need: mental stimulation
> Dinner — spaghetti & bread, neutral
> After dinner — ice cream, lonely. Real need: *companionship*

Do this for several days and notice if you reach for something specific for each emotion. Do you crave salty foods when you are bored, or do you eat whatever is most handy? What foods do you eat when angry, sad, lonely, etc.?

Knowing which emotions trigger which foods is very helpful for two reasons: First, when you become aware that you're eating because of your emotions rather than hunger, it will be easier to change that behavior. Second, when you become aware of your emotional hungers, you will be better able to meet your emotional needs in other, more constructive ways that don't involve food.

Exercise, Part 2: Creating Strategies

For whatever emotions come up, you need to create both long- and short-term ways of handling those feelings, as well as some general strategies you can use all the time. Here are some examples of the most common emotions, unmet needs, and some long- and short-term solutions.

Emotion: Boredom
Unmet need: mental stimulation
Short-term solution: read a book, watch TV
Long-term solution: go back to college for a more satisfying career

Emotion: Loneliness
Unmet need: companionship
Short-term solution: phone a friend
Long-term solution: consider dating, getting a pet, or joining some meet-up groups and finding a new hobby

Emotion: Sadness
Unmet need: someone to talk to when things don't go my way
Short-term solution: talking it over with a friend, family or clergy member
Long–term solution: taking a real hard look at what in my life is draining away my happiness; perhaps it's time to consider some changes.

You need to have several things handy you can do when these emotions comes up. So right now, think of at least five short-term things you can do when you catch yourself reaching for food when you aren't really hungry. I would recommend that these things be something you can do in less than 10 minutes, and that don't require anything you won't have readily available. If one of your solutions is "complete a puzzle," for instance, you might not be able to do it if you catch yourself emotionally eating at the office.

My list looked like this:

1) Big cold glass of water. (I recommend ice water as it will be more distracting than tap water. If I am mad, I always want something cold to cool myself off.)

2) Do something physical, like take a short walk or shoot some baskets into the trash can.
3) Do five minutes of journaling (or longer if you are really upset).
4) Take a five-minute "time out." (Remember when you were a kid and you had to do this to calm down; it works as an adult too, and sometimes just five minutes is all you need to clear your head.)
5) Read something distracting. (I recommend clicking on a fun website like www.theonion.com or www.perezhilton.com or finding stupid pet tricks on YouTube as a very healthy distraction.)

The reason why you need a list of options is because not everything will work every time. Sometimes you need to do a couple of things before the feelings pass. If for some reason they still don't pass, go ahead and allow yourself a small snack, but do it consciously by not doing anything else when you eat. The key is to stop the unconscious habit of using food to ignore our emotions, and to make eating something you do because you are physically hungry.

The "hungry meditation" listed in the next section to help you get clear about your feelings and get past the underlying issue. Most feelings will usually go away after a few minutes if you give yourself something else to do, and again, if certain emotions come up a lot, you need to start working on your long-term strategies.

Never Eat When Upset

The last and most important advice I will give on this issue; *never* ever eat when you are upset. That may seem a bit extreme, but this habit can be so destructive, it really warrants serious intervention. Even if you don't think this is your current, you don't want it to become one. If you don't follow any of my other advice, at least follow this: *Do not eat anything for at least 20 minutes following an upsetting event or episode.* This rule includes not eating even if you have a meal planned, it can wait for you to regain your peace. After 20 minutes you will have usually calmed down somewhat beyond the original upset.

Food is not your enemy, but you don't want to continue to allow it to be your friend either. Automatically eating when you are upset reinforces the idea that food is for comfort and counseling. You need to get out of the habit of making it an automatic response to being upset.

Another thing about eating when you are upset you'll likely overeat because you'll be too preoccupied to hear your body telling you to stop eating. All you will feel is the upset and often, you'll just keep eating until the strongest feelings have dissipated.

Some of you reading this may not even realize how much you have been using food in order to calm down after an upset, so I am going to warn you: creating this new habit may be harder than you think. However, this must be done so you can break the habit of reaching for food when you're upset. That will make it much easier for you to achieve your goals.

Next time you find yourself reaching for food when you aren't hungry, do the following short meditation to help you get in touch with what you are really hungry for. This meditation is based, in part on the work of hypnotherapist Michele Meiche's author of the book, *Meditations for Everyday Living*.

Hungry Meditation

Relax in a quiet place by yourself and allow your mind to go deep inside, relaxing into your inner-self. Use the deepening process from earlier in the book. When you are ready, see yourself connecting to the part of you that is hungry, the part of you that urges you to eat when you may not be physically hungry. You may feel the sense of hunger intensify as you connect more fully with this part. Now ask this part of you if it is physically hungry or if it has another need? If it is physically hungry, honor that by getting yourself something healthy to eat.

If it tells you that it's something more, ask this part of you what it's really hungry for? This part of you may give you the information in the form of pictures or in words, but carefully listen inside to what you really need. If you are not clear about what your emotional hunger is for, then ask this part for more information. Now ask "What can I give you that will better meet that need?" When it tells you how to satisfy that need, ask, "If I give you that, will you be fulfilled?" If it says "no," ask it what else it needs and keep asking until you get a clear picture of what you need to do to meet that emotional hunger.

When it says "Yes" see and feel yourself doing everything you can to meet that need. Some solutions may be short-term, like spending more time with yourself or taking a hot bath. You may also visualize long-term solutions to what's really bothering you like ending a bad relationship, but whatever it is, thank your inner self for the information and resolve to do whatever it takes to get those needs met.

Once you have a very clear idea how to meet these parts' real and deeper need, thank your inner voice for sharing the information with you, and allow yourself to come back into your fully awakened state.

Do this meditation as often as you need to until you gain a complete understanding of your real inner hunger and learn how to give yourself what you need. Often what you really need is more self-love, self-acceptance, and self-nurturing. If you did not learn how to take care of your own needs as a child, this exercise will help you get in touch with how to take care of yourself better.

Once you start observing those unmet needs and receive ideas from yourself about effective and healthy ways of handling them, you can develop short and long-term plans to manage your emotions in a way that does not involve eating.

Lesson 12: Knowing When You Are Really Done Eating

We often think about eating in terms of full and not full, but it's much healthier to just eat until you are satisfied. Often when we eat until we are "full," we have eaten so much that the body has to use too many resources to process all that food, which causes blood sugar levels to spike then crash, resulting in us becoming tired not long after we eat. If you feed yourself only enough to satisfy your appetite, you will tend to eat smaller portions more frequently and your energy level will stay more constant so you won't feel that spikes and crashes all the time. The traditional "breakfast-lunch-dinner-no snacks" model reinforces the idea that we need to eat until we're completely full, however eating smaller portions more frequently is for many people a more healthy way to eat.

Your Body Will Tell You When It's Satisfied

Now that you've started the process of paying attention to your calorie intake working on eating healthier portion sizes, and becoming aware of emotional eating, it's time to get in touch with your body's "I'm done" signals. Our bodies actually let us know when we are satisfied and don't need to continue eating, but people rarely notice or listen to that information. Iinstead they continue eating until they've finished what's on their plate, or until those around them have finished eating.

For many of us, when food became more than just sustenance we overrode our ability to notice the subtle differences between being hungry and being done because we were using food as an emotional survival tool. Even when we're call we habitually ignore the signals our bodies are trying to tell us, thus allowing ourselves to become uncomfortably full or "stuffed"." This often happens when we are eating with other people at a social event or highly distracted, like when we watch TV.

Often this habit of ignoring our natural "I'm done" signals started when we were a child. Children seem to have no trouble telling you when they are hungry and when they are finished, do they? Unfortunately, many well-intentioned parents overrode this natural ability by forcing us to stay at the table until we cleared our plates. Imagine how confusing this is to a child: your body says to stop eating but your mom and dad tell you, "you aren't done until you've finished everything in front of you." As a result we stopped trusting and listening to our own internal signals and began to use the guidance of others to let us know when we were done. Over time, listening to mom and dad caused a diminished capacity to hear our bodies own "finished" messages, and we started using the end of the plate as our stopping point.

Similarly these signals got turned off when our well-intentioned parents tried to prevent any food from being wasted. Our moms may have said, "You have to finish everything on your plate; there are starving children in Africa," or China or India, depending on what generation you grew up in. We then became confused; we were aware of the "stop eating" message, but mom is saying that this signal is wrong and that somehow children in another country will be suffering if we don't finish. The guilt over "starving children" is like a glue that keeping those feelings in place. Fast forward to the modern restaurant where a single portion size could easily feed at least two adults, and sometimes four, as a result it's doubly dangerous to keep responding to our old programming: clean your plate no matter what signals your body sends, otherwise you're guilty of wasting food and letting kids starve. In addition, if we are eating out, then we are likely visiting others, thus we're distracted from our body's signals and highly likely to eat an uncomfortable amount of food.

The key to balanced eating is relearning how to recognize and listen to your body's "done" messages. However, you may sometimes consciously override your body's "I'm done" signal when you're eating something you really enjoy. It's OK to occasionally savor something you like and to eat it for pleasure, just as long as you do it consciously by recognizing when you have had enough. Acknowledge that you are making a choice to go from satisfied to full, rather than continuing to eat until your plate is empty because that is what you were taught to do.

Foods that are low in nutritional value, like soda and chips, do not trigger very strong "not hungry anymore" signals, since they don't really give your body the physical sustenance it needs. One soda, or even 30 sodas, will never make you feel satisfied or full, and the amount of French fries that it would take to fill you up would probably make you feel sick. so you are better off trying to eat as many nutrition-filled foods as possible. I have noticed that diet soda especially seems to cause people to feel very hungry after drinking it, which often drives people to eat more food than they normally would. Empty calories (the calories in foods that have no nutritional value) really feel very empty, and often you could just keep eating those salty chips until the bag was gone without ever feeling satisfied.

Since the idea of clearing your plate and the feelings of guilt that go along with it are such a problem for many people, I have included a special meditation later in this section for just that particular issue. However, if there are other counterproductive attitudes about eating that you adopted as a child that are no longer serving you, just insert those attitudes and ideas in place of mine and that should help you overcome these issues.

What Does "I'm done" Feel Like?

Ever notice how even in a loud, crowded room, you can still pick out the voice of someone special like your child or spouse? It's because that person holds some importance to you, therefore you're attune to their voice even in a crowd. It's the same with the "I'm done" voice. Once you make the decision that this voice is important to you, you will be more attune to the signals and messages it sends you.

For some people, it's a voice that tells them they are satisfied; for others it is a general feeling of no longer being hungry. And still others tell me when they look down and see that they have eaten plenty, they know they are done. Whatever form it comes in, almost everyone tells me they get some message that tells them they're done, whether or not they always heed it. In almost all cases, the messages come in a very subtle and quiet way, almost like a whisper in your mind. But once you start noticing that whisper *and* paying attention those messages they starts to grow louder and easier to hear.

For those of you who have bodies that are conditioned to want more than is healthy, that feeling, as subtle as it is, may come after you have already eaten too much. But with time and practice, and by learning to handle your emotions in healthy ways, even that can be changed. Remember that any conditioning you received is basically a habitual response, and with effort those habits can be shifted. The following meditation will help you identify and amplify those "I'm done" feelings so that you are able to hear and respond to them more easily.

Meditation: Re-connecting with "I'm Done"

Allow yourself to relax and focus your attention inside, using *the deepening process* from earlier in the book.

When you are ready, picture yourself on a beautiful beach. It's a perfect day, there is a gentle breeze in the air, and you are feeling so at peace. Notice the waves, the way they ebb and flow, and stir the air as they crash on the beach. This is a magical place, and you feel like you can do anything. As you stroll along the beach, I want you to become aware that there is a part of you that always knows when you are satisfied because you have eaten enough food. This is the part of you that helps you eat the healthiest and most balanced amount of food and that lets you know when your body has had enough nourishment so you can stop eating before you consume too much.

Visualize this part in front of you now. You may see this part as a person or perhaps just a light, but whatever form it takes, know that it is perfect. In the past, you may have ignored this part and eaten more than you needed to but now you are beginning to realize how important this part is. As you acknowledge how important it is see this part growing bigger and noticed that its voice is getting louder. You may even see it changing form completely as it basks in your attention. Tell this part about your new goals to achieve optimal health, and that it's going to be an important part of them. Let this part know that the messages it gives you to let you know when you are done eating are very important in helping you achieve your goals and that you would like it to give you those messages in a way that is much louder and clearer than it has been in the past.

After this part lets you know that it will help you, thank it again and begin to see this part getting larger and louder. Picture a beautiful silver light coming from your throat and connecting to that part that knows when you are done, as you do this you build greater communication with this part and are able to more easily hear its messages.

Once you even more fully bonded with this part, allow yourself to drift upward, and when you are ready, open your eyes to this more complete connection with your inner-self.

Since clearing your plate is such an issue for many people, I am including an additional meditation in this lesson. It can aid you in moving past the misconception that you have to clear your plate or suffer the consequences of guilt. Do this meditation as often as you need to.

Meditation: Clear Your Plate

Allow yourself to relax and focus your attention inside. Follow your breath to go even deeper, using *the deepening process* from earlier in the book to help you relax more fully.

When you are ready, see yourself walking across a beautiful meadow. It's a gorgeous day, and it feels so peaceful in this lush green field. As you relax and enjoy the walk, I want you to think about an idea that you've carried for a long time. Whether you held it as the truth or never fully embraced it, think about the idea that you need to eat everything on your plate even if you are no longer hungry. Although the intellectual part of you knows that eating more than your body needs is not going to help you achieve your goals, on an emotional level, there may still be some resistance. Notice if there are any feelings of guilt, shame attached to your thoughts of not always eating everything on your plate. You know that you can always save anything you don't eat, or let it go back to the earth in another way. As you get more in touch with this belief, become aware of just how long you have carried it with you.

Turn around and notice that behind you there is a cord attached to this idea that you must clear your plate, and that this cord has been with you since childhood. Ask yourself if you are ready to let go of this belief and all the guilt and negative feelings that went along with it. When you feel ready, see yourself unplugging that cord the same way you would unplug a headset from your cell phone: just disconnect it and all the emotions that went along with it. Now as you disconnect this cord, watch it slither along your life's timeline to where it came from. You don't need to know when that was, but be aware that as you let it go you are freeing yourself from that belief and the emotions that went with it. Know that you are now free to throw away or save anything left on your plate after you have become satisfied and that you will no longer feel guilty for not eating it.

Once you really feel free of the belief you have to clear your plate, allow yourself to awaken and continue your day with this new flexibility.

Summary

Love your body enough to give it what it needs without giving it more than it needs. For most of us, overeating is a habit that we created a long time ago and over time we can unlearn it. When most people go on a diet, they greatly restrict their food intake to the point that their bodies feel very uncomfortable, and they end up feeling hungry. This type of dieting is neither a healthy nor wise strategy because people can usually only resist those feelings for a short while. Starting to eat less in general, while working on reconnecting with your body's "I'm done" signals, will help you create more balanced eating habits and bring awareness to eating. When you are aware of what you are doing, it's much easier to adjust it.

Lesson 13: The Purpose of Your Fat

It may be hard for some people to believe this, but you may be holding on to the fat for a reason. As humans, we do many things for reasons that we may not be consciously aware of. For instance, you may be going along on your diet and exercise program, perhaps seeing some success, and then you suddenly find yourself feeling very hungry even though you have just eaten. One thing leads to another and you abruptly give up on your diet, no longer "feel" like going to the gym, and decide that you are a failure or that you just don't have any control. However, you're not aware that there is an unconscious part of you that is making this happen because, on some level, that fat is serving a purpose in your life.

Once you understand the underlying purpose of your excess fat, you may soon recognize that it's not quite the enemy you thought it was. Often the purposes were very valid, and at one point in your life they really served you. Getting in touch with your inner-self and in order to understanding why part of you is still holding on to the fat and what purpose it serves will help you get those needs met. It will not only help you get them met, but this understanding will also enable you to establish a better connection with yourself that will help you shift other counterproductive habits.

There are many reasons why a person would, on some level, not want to let go of the fat. I will present a number of the more common ones below. See if any resonate with you.

Fat as protection: This is probably the most common purpose I see with my clients. Like a comfortable coat, a layer of fat can feel almost like a buffer between you and a world that doesn't always feel safe. This is particularly true for women who have been a victim of any kind of physical or sexual abuse. There can be an unconscious feeling that being fat might make you less attractive to predators and act as insulation from physical harm.

Unfortunately, being fat and physically unhealthy in general is more likely to make you a victim than to keep you safe. If this is an issue for you, consider doing things that would actually make you safe, like taking a self-defense class or increasing your awareness of your surroundings and paying attention to what you are doing. Better yet, listen to your own internal warning signs that something or someone is not right. Often this is the best defense you could ever have, and you would be wise to listen to it.

A great excuse: Sometimes there are difficult events or situations in our lives that could help us achieve our life goals, then being fat gives us a great excuse for not following through with our plans, or for not even trying in the first place. When confronted with these situations or events (public speaking, dating, a job opportunity), we're armed with a ready-made excuse, "I should wait until I lose___ pounds before I do that." or when we try and don't succeed "This, that, or the other didn't happen because I am fat." I coached a client who worked in public relations and was afraid of expanding her business into a new area and being overweight made a great excuse. Her belief was, "I can't go for the bigger jobs unless I lose the weight. No one wants to hire an overweight public relations person in the entertainment industry." It turns out she was also afraid that if she did lose weight, she would get so much business, she wouldn't have any time for herself. On some level it felt better to be fat and have free time than deal with the hassles that come with greater success.

I loved using fat as an excuse. It was the reason for every job I didn't get, every relationship that didn't work out, and every snub I ever got. And on some level it made life easier because it meant I never had to be personally responsible for my failures. Giving up the fat meant giving up the mother of all excuses and a part of me really fought letting that go.

If this is an issue for you, know this: you can't run from problems, fears, and difficult situations-they only get louder and bigger. When there is something you can do about your issues, then do it, as in the case of my client in the PR industry, who really only needed an assistant so she could handle more business. If there isn't anything you can do, then you have to let it go and just work harder to accomplish your goals. You can do anything, but you have to start by letting go of the excuses.

To avoid getting into relationships: I see this excuse a lot with both women and men who are single and who for various reasons do not want to date. What they tell me is that having to say "no" makes them so uncomfortable that they would rather people didn't find them attractive. I worked with a woman who was a widow and still going through the grieving process. She started to get nervous as she began to lose weight because she really didn't want to be asked out on dates yet. The reality is that when you are overweight, being asked out on dates doesn't happen as often and part of you knows it and may not want to let go of the fat for that reason.

When you are ready to date again, you will know it; and if you decide never to date again after the loss of a partner or after a traumatic breakup, that's OK too. Respect yourself enough to not succumb to pressure from family, friends, or society and date only when *you* are ready. Sometimes giving yourself permission to wait is sometimes all you need in order to let go of the weight and to help you create a healthy body.

Fitting in with family: Many people have observed that overweight parents often have overweight kids. Nutritionists sometimes say it's because the kids picked up their parents' bad habits, but I don't think that's the whole story. People want to fit in with their family and being different can be very uncomfortable. If you are in a family full of fat people it might feel very isolating to be the lone thin person, so you adopt the family "norm" and do what you need to in order to look like everyone else. This can sometimes be reinforced by the expectation that you'll always be fat like everyone else in your family. If you expect to be fat like your mom, you will literally grow into that expectation. I have even seen clients who were uncomfortable losing weight because weight loss success meant leaving some people behind. The concern is if you succeed where everyone else failed, will those same people still love you?

If the fear of no longer fitting in with family is an issue for you, it's usually because you aren't fitting in with them in other ways as well. To some extent you may just have to accept that and move on. We are born into our families, and unlike our friends, we don't get to chose them, so we have to acknowledge and accept that we may not be like them in every way. The key is to not let those feelings or fears prevent you from having the life you want and deserve. You may actually find that as you get healthy, you become an example for your family of how to create a new better health for themselves.

Fat gets you attention: In a perfect family, every person would get as much attention and love as they need, but as we all know, that is often not the case. Sometimes becoming fat, or any other self-created health problem, like an eating disorder or drug use, can be an unconscious attempt to elicit much-needed attention and love. Even negative attention can feel good to someone who feels isolated and lonely. For example, at one of my very first jobs, the office manager who hired me was kind, fun, and capable, but she also weighed over 350 pounds was very plain looking and it didn't take long to learn that everyone in the office made fun of her for her weight. One day over coffee she let it slip that she knew how much people laughed at her, and I asked her how she felt about it. She said something I will never forget: "I know I am not pretty, but if I wasn't fat would anyone notice me at all?" That was so sad, but I understood that with that circle of people it was probably true. She was so unique and special, but because she only saw herself as fat and she relished the attention she got for it; for someone who is very lonely, even bad attention provides some attention.

I suggest that if you need some attention in your life, then I suggest that you look inot some of the many healthy ways of getting it. For instance, you can take an acting class, singing lessons, or dancing lessons—anything where you are putting yourself out there in a creative way.

Rebelling: Using your weight as a method of rebellion often starts as a child; especially for those who had parents that placed too much importance on physical appearance. All the same I come across this issue with clients whose spouses are not meeting their needs or whose spouses are belittling them for being overweight. How motivating is it really when someone says, "You need to lose weight. I'm not finding you as attractive anymore because you are overweight"? A part of us will always feel like we should be loved no matter what and we will we hold on to the fat for that reason.

If there is an element of rebellion in the purpose of your fat, you may want to ask yourself if losing weight and getting healthier is something you want for you. If it's not, that's OK; you can always start trying to lose weight again when it is. But unless you truly want to be healthy and lose weight for *yourself*, it's very difficult to get motivated to do all the things you need in order to achieve your goal.

Fat as a way of handling secrets: I love Suze Orman. In her show she often talks about how people put on weight when they have secret debt. I agree with her 100%, though debt is not the only secret that we hide behind fat. People have all kinds of secrets they conceal with fat, including ongoing abuse, feelings of unhappiness, and family lies such as "Dad didn't die; he's in prison." These kinds of secrets can cause us to put on fat as a way of hiding from a life we aren't completely happy with.

If keeping secrets is keeping you fat, then it's time to let those secrets come out of your body. You don't have to share them with anyone unless you want to, but you do need to draw them outside of yourself by journaling, telling them to a friend with whom you are comfortable, or talk to a counselor if you need support. However you do it, they have to come out, and you have to acknowledge how you feel, at the very least be sure that you acknowledge your secrets to yourself. When you start sharing, you will be shocked to find out how many people you know have had those same experiences, and you won't feel so alone with them anymore.

There are many reasons someone might hold on to fat, and I have listed just the most common ones I have seen with clients. It's important to be aware that the part of you that is holding on to the fat does have a real reason and purpose. When you begin to really look at your reasons, I want you to do so with a loving heart. The part that's been holding on to the fat has been trying to help you in some way. Unfortunately that purpose is also interfering with your higher purpose of losing weight. Regardless, it's important to at least acknowledge that your reasons for being fat are valid.

The following meditation will help you connect with your personal reasons for holding on to the fat as well as well as to help you devise healthier ways of getting those needs met. This meditation is based, in part on the work of hypnotherapist Michele Meiche's author of the book, *Meditations for Everyday Living*.

This process is about understanding the "why" behind the "what" of your current body situation. As you do this meditation, try to go through the steps without judgment about what comes up. Just continue even if the information given doesn't make a lot of sense.

Meditation: Healing Reasons for Holding on to Fat

Find a quiet place in your home where you will not be disturbed for a few minutes. Sit comfortably in a chair or on the ground and close your eyes. Allow yourself to relax as you focus your attention more fully on the inside using *the deepening process* from earlier in the book.

When you are ready, imagine yourself on a beautiful sandy beach. You are there to meet a very important part of yourself. This is the part of you that is holding on to the body fat, and it has a purpose. See this part in front of you now, and when you are ready, embrace this part and send it love. Remember, this part has been trying to help you even if what it was doing created different challenges for you.

Now in your own words ask this part, "Why am I holding on to the fat?" It may give you an answer in pictures or feelings, but whatever it does, make a mental note of it, thank it for sharing, and when you are ready, ask, "What purpose does the fat serve?" It may give you a different answer this time, or it may be the same, but either way thank it for what it's been doing for you and send it love.

Now think about all the things this part was trying to achieve by holding on to the fat, and as you relax and go a little deeper, imagine all the other ways you can meet those needs. Visualize how you could bring those ways of being into your life, and resolve to do some of them right away.

When you feel you have all the information you need, as well as a new strategy, open your eyes. Figure out a way to bring those ideas into your life right now, knowing that this information could be the key to your weight-loss journey.

I suggest doing this meditation several times. You may find that the first time you do it you don't get all the information you need or that the purpose part of you may be unwilling to let go of what it has been doing for you, but don't give up. Keep in mind, this is the first time you have even acknowledged this part of you, and there may be some initial resistance to hearing what it has to say, but with practice you will be able to get it right. Love yourself enough to take the time that you and this part of you needs.

Now that you have the information on both the purpose of your fat and how you can get those needs met in other ways, it's very important that you follow through on the strategies you created in this meditation. Think about what changes you need to make in your life so that the purpose your fat was serving so that your goals can be met in a different way. If you had trouble coming up with a strategy, do the process again or refer to the ones I listed earlier in this section.

Summary:

Once you understand that your fat had a purpose, it's much easier to handle getting those needs met in a healthy way.

The key is that you need to work with your inner-self rather than against it in order to achieve your highest goals. Love yourself enough to acknowledge your needs and take steps to get those needs met. The payoff is well worth the effort.

Lesson 14: The Saboteur

If fat is serving any purpose in your life, the inner saboteur is making sure that the fat stays right where it is no matter what. You know the part I am talking about, its the part of you that makes cookies taste *so* good when you have just gone on a diet, that makes you feel hungry just after you've eaten, that makes crunchy potato chips sound like manna from the gods, and a slice of cake something you must have right now or you are going to die. The saboteur comes up with all kinds of excuses and reasons for why you can't work out right now or do whatever else you should be doing to lose weight. You may have every good intention of losing weight, but the saboteur is like a computer program running in the background that derails all of your diet and exercise plans. And like other parts of your personality, this part does not like change because that requires you to step out of the old groove and create new habits. And since 90% of our daily activities are habit-based, that means making some big internal changes.

Clients often ask me, "So how do I get rid of this part?" Well, not only can you not just "get rid of it," but you wouldn't want to even if you could. Consider this; your saboteur has been incredibly successful at helping you fail to lose weight. For some, it's managed to interfere with your best efforts for your entire life. It's proven that it can do a very good job when given this task. If you had an employee who was that effective and you no longer wanted them working on a specific project you wouldn't be foolish enough to let them go, would you? No, instead you would reassign them to a different project.

Many of us have created a very adversarial relationship with our saboteur, so much so that the part of us that wants to be thin seems to really hate the part of us that interferes with that. But these are both parts of our personality, and as such they both have their valid purposes. The key here is to stop hating the saboteur (after all its part of you), connect and make friends with it, and reassign it to projects that'll help you achieve your goals.

The best way to connect with your inner saboteur is through meditation. The meditation below will help you get in touch with this part and give it a more life affirming job.

Exercise: Finding New Tasks for the Saboteur

Before you do this meditation, take a few moments to ponder the following question: "If I could give the saboteur another task that would actually help me lose weight, what would that be?" Repurposed saboteurs can make great finders, so you may want to consider asking it to point out things that will help you achieve your goals. For example, you might assign it to:

- Remind you to exercise or help you find physical activities you like doing.
- Help you get excited about healthier foods or finding new recipes.
- Encourage you to stick to your new healthy eating programs.

Meditation: Saboteur to Friend

Find a quiet place to relax, focus your attention inside, and use the deepening process from earlier in the book to help you go even deeper.

When you are ready, see yourself walking though a beautiful meadow. It's a warm sunny day, and you feel very peaceful enjoying your stroll in this lush green landscape. You have come to this place to meet a very important part of your personality. This is the part that in the past has been interfering with your efforts to create the healthiest body possible for you. In the past you may have been angry with the saboteur but now you have a new understanding and appreciation for how powerful it really is. You understand on a deep level that this part of you had a purpose and may have actually thought it was helping you in some way.

Ask the saboteur to stand before you now. You may visualize this part as looking like you, or perhaps it will just be a light, but whatever it looks like, be sure to send it love.

Acknowledge that this part has been very skilled at what it's been doing, and ask it, "What is your purpose?" or "Why are you doing this?" As you allow this part of you to fully communicate it may give you the answers in the form of pictures, words, or even just a feeling as you allow this part to really tell you what it's been doing. If you don't completely understand what it's showing you, ask for clarification and continue asking until you are very clear about what its purpose is.

When it gives you an answer, embrace the inner saboteur part and thank it for what it's been doing, acknowledging that it has a very noble purpose. Let this part know that it was been doing a tremendous job for you, but now you are releasing it from this task and giving it a new, more important one. See, hear, and feel yourself letting this part of you know about your goals and what you want to create with your body and your health. You can share pictures, feelings, or words, whichever you prefer, knowing this part will fully understand what you are sharing.

When you are ready, assign the now former saboteur the new task of helping you achieve your goals. If you have specific things you would like it to do for you, communicate those now. Let your new friend really understand how you want it to help you and that you would like it to fully commit to your goals just as you have. Tell it that because this task is so important, you are putting your former saboteur on the job since it's already proven it can is very good at getting things done. Let this part really see how much you appreciate it and how important this new job is.

When you feel you have fully expressed yourself and that your new friend is committed, embrace it and then send it on its way—it has much work to do.

When you feel complete, open your eyes and continue with your day.

Summary

You may notice over the course of the day, or the next few days, that you start getting ideas about what you can do to achieve your goals. When you do get insights or inspirational flashes, acknowledge that your former saboteur is hard at work helping you achieve your goals. Use your journal to record any of these insights and inspirations as well as feelings that come up for you. This journey can be emotional, so don't be afraid if not–so-happy feelings come up as well. This is a physical and emotional journey. The more you practice these new ideas, the more information you will receive. Pay attention to the information your new friend is sharing with you. It just may send you the key that makes all your health and wellness dreams come true.

Lesson 15: Your Weight-Gain Trigger

If you were able to plot someone's weight on one side of a chart and a timeline of all their major life challenges on the other, you would find that the most significant weight gains happened soon after or during a very difficult patch in that person's life. I hear a lot from clients: "I was going through a divorce and my life was in a general state of chaos." "I had just lost my job...." "It started when my husband died..." Followed with, "Everything else seemed more important to me than my body, and before I knew it, I was 60 pounds heavier."

if they really think about it almost everyone can come up with a single event or series of events that triggered the current state of their body. Typically, weight gain is triggered by major life changes, like the start or end of a relationship, marriage, divorce, the birth of a child, death of a loved one, loss of a job or business, or other major financial crisis. For me it started with puberty and the unhappiness of my teenage years, which got worse with each succeeding upset in my life.

It's important to mention that I do not include pregnancy on the list of most common weight-gain triggers since your body is supposed to gain weight during this time as part of being healthy. However, if after a year you haven't dropped back down to within a few pounds of your pre-baby weight, then it could be more than just physical. I have worked with women who gained more weight in the year after having a child than they did during their pregnancy, often as a result of overeating due to postpartum depression or stresses relating to this major life change.

I would have to say the most common weight gain trigger I see for women is being in an unhealthy or unsatisfying relationship. In fact, this is often the first question I ask when I meet a new female client, "How is your relationship with your boyfriend, husband, or partner?" This usually catches people off guard because they expect me to ask about their diet. The diet is interesting, but no matter what they are eating if they are in my office I already know they are eating too much of it.

For men, the most common trigger I see is job or business loss, including the loss of prestige in a job, getting demoted, or losing out on a promotion opportunity.

But for both sexes, money is a huge trigger. As mentioned before, Suze Orman talks a lot in her TV show (*The Suze Orman Show*), about health and wealth being connected, and I have often seen those two issues tied together a lot in my practice. The loss of a job, business, or money in the stock market, and the resulting possible loss of a house and the incurring of credit card debt, are all major reasons why people start eating too much.

Basically, when some part of our lives gets out of balance, we overeating to compensate, and thus we gain weight. Relationship trouble, poor finances, or dealing with grief or other major life changes stirs up emotions and causes great chaos. These events may also make us feel out of control and uncertain of how to get that control back. It doesn't matter if our lives really are out of control, if we feel that we cannot effectively cope with our feelings about what is going on. That's when we might turn to food as a way to change how we feel. It's also a way of feeling comforted in times of upset and it also provides a good distraction.

Acknowledging and Letting Go of Blame

Usually when people really look at what caused their most recent weight gain they experience feelings of blame, both toward the self and others. It is especially hard for people to accept responsibility for something they clearly did to themselves, like eating too much and putting on excessive weight. But blaming other people or situations part of the glue that keeps the situation in place, because in essence it's saying, "You have to change or I won't be able to." The problem with blame is that it gives away your personal power to something outside you, and let's face it, the fast food restaurants are not going to stop serving unhealthy food just because you need to lose some weight.

You have to be so committed to losing weight and being healthy that you won't let anyone or anything get in your way. That starts by making the decision to take responsibility for creating your body's current state of health and seizing this opportunity to fix it.

I know I blamed everyone and everything for my weight and spent a lot of time and energy being angry. I blamed parents, kids at school, models, and McDonalds for seducing me with hot apple pies and French fries, but most importantly, I blamed myself.

What's interesting about self-blame is that it amounts to the part of you that longs to be thin blaming and being angry with the part of you that's not. If you think about it, the whole idea of blaming yourself—getting mad at parts of yourself—is really ridiculous. That internal blame just leads to conflict, and just like conflicts at work don't help get the job done, conflicts in yourself can really interfere with your success.

In reality, I was far from powerless and could have made significant changes to my eating and exercise habits much earlier in my life, but I chose instead to focus on blame and missed opportunities to change, mostly because I wasn't ready to take responsibility for my actions. However, when I was ready to step on the scale, look at how I got there, and acknowledge my own personal power to change anything I wanted, then my body and my life really did change in some very significant ways.

When you can shift out of the blame state and start really looking at how you got to this place, then you can devise powerful solutions that will help you create the life you want. Give yourself the gift of letting go of the habit of blame and the blindness it fosters, and instead embrace truth and reclaim the change-making abilities it offers. Here is a list of some of the specific agents in your life that you'll need to stop blaming for your weight problem:

Blaming family: I will be the first to admit that family can make it very hard to have the life you want. But once you become an adult and move away from home you have the power to set boundaries and let them know what you need. Later, I will discuss how to handle an unsupportive family, but for now, consider letting go of blaming them for what happened.

Genetics: Related to blaming family, I often hear clients say they believe they got "fat genes" from their parents. Many of those same clients feel like that renders their weight-loss efforts hopeless. The truth is that genetics is a very small factor in whether a person will be overweight or not. For the most part, if your parents were overweight and you became overweight, it's mostly because you on some level wanted to fit in with your family or just adopted their eating and exercise habits.

Fast food: It's clear that fast food restaurants are more concerned with profits than with our health, but that's not really a secret, is it? It's not their fault you ate too much of their very fattening foods—it's yours. So resolve to make better/healthier choices in the future.

Models: Clients often report that they blame models for making them feel bad about themselves, but that would be like blaming Tiger Woods for making all other golfers look bad. If you want to achieve optimal health you have to stop blaming and hating that which you secretly admire. Rather, try to appreciate all the hard work and discipline that goes into creating the body and life you want. Models are people doing a job just like you, and, trust me, if you had the same financial incentive to stay in shape, you could probably stick to a diet too.

Blaming society in general: While it's true that the world *should* treat everyone the same regardless of their weight, the fact is that, it doesn't. It's not right, but we will drive ourselves crazy if we let every fat joke we hear upset us. A wise person once told me that when you stop caring about what people say, the bullies will stop saying anything bad because it won't be fun for them anymore.

Blaming yourself: Taking responsibility isn't about blaming yourself for what happened. That's done; it's in the past. This is about acknowledging that you put yourself into this situation and about learning from your past mistakes so you can get back to optimal health. If you can't take personal responsibility for your health, it's very difficult to feel empowered enough to make the necessary changes to be free.

Forgive Yourself for Letting This Happen

Ultimately, you have to forgive yourself for letting your body reach such an unhealthy state: for not eating less food when you started putting on too much weight, for not exercising enough, and for not loving yourself enough to do all the things you need to do in order to keep your body healthy. But, most importantly, you need to forgive yourself for being so critical and so hard on yourself about the fact that this happened.

For the purposes of weight loss, forgiveness begins with acknowledging how you got here, and then letting go of the feelings of hurt, anger, and resentment you have toward *yourself* about your current state of health and how you got there. Next, you must decide to let those feelings be in the past as you move toward a future free of feelings of guilt and upset over it. Ultimately, it's about removing the label of being a fat person and permanently getting rid of the "fat section" of your closet and just having your "clothing section" full of wonderful clothes for the body you love.

If there are others who have contributed to your current state of health by being unkind, unloving, unsupportive, and perhaps even cruel in their words or actions, the process of forgiveness is *not* about saying what they did was OK. It wasn't. In this case, forgiveness is about releasing the hurt so that you can move past those feelings and into a place of health without dragging the past behind you like an anchor.

If you are someone who became overweight as a result of something *not* within your control, such as through cancer treatment recovery, a thyroid problem, or other medical condition that caused weight gain; you may still have a lot of anger toward yourself and toward the illness or the doctors or anyone or anything else you think might be responsible. If that is the case for you, I would encourage you to still do this exercise since it is about acknowledging what happened and moving past that place into a new, healthier way of being.

Exercise: Acknowledging Weight-Gain Triggers

I want you to spend some time thinking about and writing down what triggered your most recent weight gain. If you have gained and lost weight many times, try to recall what triggered each of those incidents so you can be aware of what causes you to eat more food than you need. For many people, this has been an up and down battle: weight goes up in times of stress and challenge and down in times of calm and peace.

While it's not essential to know which situations or upsets got you to this place now, it is very helpful to know your triggers, so you can really try to piece together what life events caused your weight gain. As I mentioned before, since it's usually major life upsets that trigger weight gain, start by looking through the timeline of your life for relationship challenges and job/business troubles. As money creates issues for both sexes, also look at your tax returns for the past few years and review the times of financial troubles. Again its not essential but helpful to know what kinds of life challenges cause you to overeat since its very likely the same or similar situation may come up again later in life and you want to be prepared with a plan for handling your emotions that does not involve food.

If you are like me and have never been your ideal weight in your adult life, think about what was going on in your childhood that caused you to eat more than you needed. Make a mental note of any blame you may feel toward yourself or others for contributing to this situation. There may indeed be real things others did that contributed to this issue, but continuing to blame them only takes your power away. Eventually, you'll need to let go of the blame game and step into your power to make changes and have the life you want.

Meditation: Forgiveness

Find a quiet place where you can relax undisturbed. Allow your breath to bring you deep inside, using *the deepening process* from earlier in the book to help you go even deeper.

Picture yourself walking along a path in the forest and you come upon a small house with a big door. Go inside and notice that it's a large empty room with a small fire burning in the center. Move closer to the fire and notice that it has a brilliant blue healing flame. Allow yourself to absorb the healing energy and light from this flame.

As you stand there before the flame, think about all the things you did that contributed to your current state of physical health. Think of the habits, like overeating and not exercising that made it hard for your body to be its healthiest. Create pictures in your mind that represent these behaviors and visualize them in front of you. Now pour all your feelings about how those habits affected you into those pictures, pulling all the associated feelings out of your body and putting the energy from them into the pictures. When you are ready, drop those pictures into the fire and watch the flames getting higher and brighter as you burn away those old habits. Feel the fire getting warmer as it releases the energy trapped in those pictures.

Now I want you to create pictures that represent all the blame you feel toward yourself and others about your weight. Picture any mean or belittling statements people made or actions that were unsupportive and pour your feelings into those pictures. Make the images as dark and as big as they need to be to fully represent those feelings. As you fill your images in with your emotions, allow yourself to feel relieved as you release these emotions from your body and soon your body will feel free and blameless. Since you are now free of your former non-supportive habits and blame, allow yourself to take a deep breath and experience life as being lighter and more free.

Now in this special magical place, acknowledge that mistake and failures don't exist, they are only learning opportunities. Continue letting go of all the feelings and bad memories that you have about these situations and events as you see the healing flame consume all of those upsets. Feel cleansed, refreshed, and free—free of the past hurts and upsets, and free to create the body you want.

Now step outside the house and fill your mind with the images that represent your new habits and ways of being that will take you to your healthiest body. Create another image that represents the new level of self-love and acceptance that you will be bringing into your life. See yourself continuing on your life's path, leaving the past behind and taking your new ways of being with you.

When you are ready, open your eyes and enjoy these new feelings.

Summary

Blame is like sticky glue that can keep your old habits and old body in place. Letting go of the blame and of past missteps, as well as releasing others of blame for your health issues is a big step toward detaching yourself from that old body and embracing the healthiest version of you. Love yourself enough to do that work.

Lesson 16: Who Is There for You?

It would be nice to say that everyone in your life is always going to be 100% behind you and supportive. But one of the hardest life lessons a person ever has to learn is that some of the people closest to you, including your own family, not want you to succeed and may even try to sabotage your efforts. Whether it's your best friend, your family, your boyfriend/girlfriend, or colleagues, these people can really make you second guess yourself and interfere with your intention of creating the life you want. And the most difficult part is often that you may never understand their reasons. I see this all the time in my practice, and it came up a lot for me when I was losing weight.

These behaviors sometimes show up as sly unsupportive comments to the effect that what you are doing isn't working because you are still fat, or as gifts of special food from a loved one who knows you are on a diet, or what I think is the most unsupportive of all; a refusal to financially support the project of losing weight even when there are resources available. For instance, a spouse may complain about having to pay for a gym membership that will help you improve your health, the higher grocery bill because fresh fruits and veggies cost more, any increased medical costs, or even the cost of new running shoes. Usually these are followed by comments or reminders of all the other times money was spent, and you either failed to lose weight, or you did and then gained it back. In my experience, these are all complaints that hide the fact that on some level the person making them really doesn't want you to lose weight.

In my case, my mother was the least supportive family member, and that showed up in some subtle and passive-aggressive ways. For example, after I had lost 60 pounds and told her I had to buy new all new clothes replacing even underwear and bra's she said, "So sad, you had such lovely clothes, and now you have to buy all new ones. Such a waste." The battered woman's shelter that got all my plus-sized office clothing did not think it was a waste and neither did I. Her comments came after a lifetime of her saying, "Oh, when you lose weight you can buy this, do that, etc.," so I had expected her to be happy for me, but instead it seemed she was not. That incident reminded me that this was not the first time it had happened. In fact, there were many times growing up when I had tried to lose weight and my mother would be so concerned about the cost of buying new clothes that she did not encourage my efforts in any way. For instance, when I was 11 years old and rather chubby, my doctor told my mother not to worry about me weight, that the only thing I needed to do was enroll in some kind of sport. I was excited when he said that because I had always wanted to, but my mother didn't want to drive me to practice, so I could never go. I suspected that because she had struggled with her own weight her whole life, the idea that I might succeed where she had failed made her uncomfortable.

For most people the most unsupportive person in their life is their spouse. Unlike a girlfriend or boyfriend you can just stop hanging out with, you have to deal with your spouse's interference (unsupportive behaviors) every day. What I hear most often is that the husband says he is afraid that if his wife loses weight she will look so much more attractive than him and that will leave him. I had a client who had been married for 35 years tell me, "He's so insecure. He thinks I will start looking so good I will leave him for someone better than him. I've lived with him, raised his kids, and done his laundry for over 35 years. Why would I leave him because I lost weight?"

Sometimes manipulative behaviors can be disguised as supportive behaviors. I once worked with a woman who, after having a child at the age of 40, found it difficult to lose the baby weight. When she told her husband about her plan to lose 50 pounds, he very excitedly promised her that when she did, he would take her on a cruise. It sounded nice at first, however it was just a manipulative ploy to try to get her to lose weight. When they got married two years earlier, she had wanted to go on a cruise for their honeymoon, but because of money issues they hadn't gone. Ever since then, they had saved enough money and had been working on plans to go. However, instead of supporting her weight loss efforts he told her that her weight was making him find her very unattractive. She was already feeling severely depressed about her weight, and now her husband was telling her that he would only take her on a cruise if she got down to 135 pounds (her high school weight). So, the promised reward of going on a cruise turned out to be a manipulative and destructive ploy to try to get her to lose weight. In reality, they didn't need a cruise; they needed marriage counseling to heal their relationship.

Your spouse is not the only one who can try to interfere with your plans for a healthier life. Coworkers and jealous friends can also undermine your efforts. People don't like to admit it, but when it comes to group dynamics, everyone seems to prefer the status quo. When you are the overweight friend in a group and you start to lose weight, others may begin to feel threatened. Women in particular are socialized to see other successful females as competition.

As you change your life and become healthier, people in your life will have to adjust to the new you as much as you will. For some people that adjustment can be very difficult and might bring up insecurities they have. However, you can't let someone else's issues interfere with your plans for a healthier you. Think of losing weight as a part of a bigger plan for having a better life. If you let someone interfere with this part of your life, they will eventually interfere with every part of your life and you won't be happy with the results of that.

Until you are clear about how supportive or unsupportive someone will be, it's best not to share your plans with him or her. I know it sounds secretive, but think of it as protecting yourself and your new growth, until your new habits and ways of being are firmly in place. Love yourself enough to know and acknowledge where people really stand with you and what roles they can play in supporting your higher plans. That doesn't mean not spending time with them if you want to, but maybe you just don't share everything with them until you really know if they will truly be on your side.

The other part of this is to decide for yourself if someone's behavior is supportive or not. Lots of people will say, "Wow, I am so happy for you," and then follow it with "Do you think you will succeed this time?" which at first glance might sound OK, but it's really not because it reminds you of your past failures rather than reinforcing your future success. Other times the behavior will come in the form of actions. I had a boyfriend who offered to go jogging with me, but only because, as he informed me, "You go too slow. I will keep the pace up so you can lose weight faster," which to me always sounded kind of condescending.

The bottom line in deciding if someone is being supportive is sensing how it *feels*. If you hang around someone and at the end of it you feel tired and worse about yourself than before you started, then their behavior is not supportive regardless of the person's intent. It's all about how it feels for you, and being honest with yourself is what you really need for this process to work.

Exercise: Who Is There for You?

First, make a list of the people who have the most influence in your life right now and honestly rate them on their supportiveness of what you are doing. Key word; *honestly*. You need to be honest at least with yourself if no one else. How supportive is your mom *really*.

Now this isn't about judging your mother or grandma, although you may find that when you look at you list you start getting mad. This exercise is about being more aware of what is going on in your life right now and what impact certain people are on you. If you won't admit to yourself that your husband's comments about your backside are not helping you feel better about yourself, who will you be honest with? Your list might look like this:

> Boyfriend — supportive
> Mom — unsupportive
> Brother — somewhat supportive

Dad — unsupportive
Friend Cara — extremely supportive
Friend Jackleen — very supportive
Friend Richard — very supportive
Coworker Jane — unsupportive
Grandma — very unsupportive
Friend Tia — very supportive

The second part of this exercise is figuring out how you are going to handle your family and friends now that you are acknowledging their words aren't supportive. I actually had to be honest with my father about the impact of what he was saying. One day my dad said, "Jill, it's great you are losing weight, and maybe now that you are thinner you can get a husband." I got very angry when he said this because he clearly believed that my weight was the only reason for the other "problem" he thought I had. To my father and grandmother, being a 30 year old woman and still single made me an old maid, and their feelings had a detrimental impact on me. I calmly reminded my dad that I was very healthy, and that when I was overweight I had two marriage proposals that I decided to turn down, so weight was clearly not the reason why I was single. And, most importantly, I told him, "Dad, those kinds of statements don't help. I know you mean well, but I would rather not talk about my weight, good or bad, anymore."

He was quite surprised. Since then, other than saying I looked good after I lost weight, he's never really made any other comments on my weight, and this has helped my relationship with my father tremendously. I also had to stop talking about weight with my mother and grandmother as those conversations always seemed to go badly for similar reasons.

Sometimes the best strategy for dealing with unsupportive family members and friends is to spend less time with them or to direct the conversations away from talk of your weight. Other times your best strategy is to tell them their comments on food, your diet, or health don't help you lose weight. But perhaps the best strategy of all is simply to spend more time with someone who is more supportive of you, or even just spend more time supporting yourself. Whatever strategy you decide is best for handling your family and friends, I suggest you think about it now so that you are prepared for the next time someone makes a very unsupportive jab like "You are very pretty. If you would only lose some weight...."

When it comes to people who are supportive of you and your efforts, consider having them take a more active role in your life and being part of what I call your "Wellness Team". There are few major projects that get done without the help of a team, and this is especially true of losing weight. I recommend creating a team consisting of supportive friends and at least one wellness practitioner that you see regularly to help you achieve your goals. My Wellness Team included a personal trainer, a chiropractor, a hypnotherapist, and my good friend Cara who were always on my side, encouraging me along the way. You don't need to tell them they are part of your Wellness Team—they may think that's weird, like you just enrolled them in a club. It's a matter of planning on doing more things like spending more time with them.

    I found my personal trainer to be most helpful because she had worked with many other people with similar goals, and when I struggled she was always there to remind me that I would have weight loss success. In a way my personal trainer became the supportive family member I wished I had. With family who may have seen you try and fail many times, there could be an expectation that this time will be like the others. Someone who hasn't seen that history doesn't have that expectation, and this can be very helpful and supportive. Also, unlike my family who tended to like things to stay the same and didn't really want me to succeed, she was highly invested in my success, and I found this very helpful.

    I have said before that losing weight is an emotional journey, and it really is in more ways than one. As you lose weight and heal some of the emotional issues that caused you to gain it in the first place, there will be some ups and downs. In addition, as your body burns through the fat, it almost feels like you are burning through old emotions as well, because there will be times when you will be confronted with an ugly memory from your past and all the emotions that went with it. Rather than stuffing away those feelings with food, you will need to be there for yourself when they come up and sometimes seek outside support if needed. For example, I worked with an amazing hypnotherapist who helped me handle the emotional part of the process, and several talented personal trainers for the physical aspects of it.

If resources are limited, at the very least I recommend joining a Weight Watchers group or something like it. Weight Watchers is an inexpensive yet supportive program and I have found their facilitators to be both helpful and caring. You can also look for meet-Up groups of people like yourself who are on the path to achieving optimal health.

The people you find to be part of your personal support group can be worth their weight in gold, so to speak, because they can motivate you and support you in ways that might at times be hard to generate within yourself.

Exercise: Creating Your Wellness Team

Make a list of at least five people currently in your life that can be part of your Wellness Team and what each of their roles would be. See my example below:

> Chiropractor: to provide nutritional advice and keep my back in shape while I do more physical exercise.
> Personal trainer: to work out two days a week and to give me new exercises to move my program forward.
> Hypnotherapist: to help me create healthy habits and anchor those on a deep level.
> Group exercise teacher: to kick my butt at the 5:45am Tues. & Thurs. class
> Friend Jackleen: to meet for a hike at least once a week for a workout and chick chat.
> My dog Spot: to take on a long walk twice a day; maybe he could use a jog, too.

Next, enroll some of people on your Wellness Team by telling them about your goals and asking them for their help. However, remember my advice about not telling people who you are unsure about, only sharing with those that are on your team. You may find your personal trainer, chiropractor, naturopath, or medical doctor have a lot of great information about things you can do to make your dreams a reality. Your dog might not respond to your plans, but he or she will probably be enthusiastic about the increased exercise, and that can be very helpful. Most people would actually love to help you. You just have to ask.

Summary

It's very important that you be honest with yourself about who is and who isn't really there for you, because your unsupportive friends and family members can truly make achieving your goals more difficult than it has to be. By contrast, spending time with and being supported by those who really are on your side can make all the difference in whether you succeed or fail.

Lesson 17: Self-Love, Self-Respect, and Putting Yourself First

Long ago I made a choice I could either love myself or hate myself. I choose love and I like the results of that. When you love yourself, you make better choices.

———

Queen
Latifah

Now that we have gotten clear about who is and who is not there for you, it's important to connect to your most valuable supportive asset—you. Whenever someone asks me what the key to losing weight is I always tell them two things: 1) there are really lots of *keys* to losing weight and creating optimal health for yourself, and you may have to use them all; and 2) love, self–love, and self-respect. Love is the anchor that enables you to do everything necessary for optimal health. Love gets you up in the morning to go to the gym because you love your body enough to want to keep it strong. Love tells you to pass on the chips and eat vegetables because you want to keep your body-temple healthy and free of junk. Love enables you to respect and take care of your own needs first. Love gives you the courage to say "no" to people and situations that are not in your best interests, even when it might create conflict. Love, self-love, and self-acceptance make all things possible.

I can honestly tell you that this was the toughest lesson I had to learn as part of my journey. Until I started working on it, I was never able to feel self-love, and it's no wonder when I think about my childhood. At a very young age I was taught that loving yourself was "selfish," that asking for something for yourself when our family didn't have a lot of money was "greedy." Sharing ideas that went against my family's core values resulted in you being loudly told "you are wrong." But worst of all, I learned that at any moment my body could be the recipient of my father's inability to control his anger. No wonder I never learned about self-love; no one in my life showed me how. As a result, I found that respecting my body and loving myself is very much a learned skill.

Many of my clients tell me the same thing: they truly can't seem to access feelings of self-love and, accordingly, don't treat themselves with the respect they truly want and deserve. They do not put themselves first, they put bad food in their bodies; they talk down to themselves; and they do things they don't want to do because they were taught one of their roles was to please others.

Getting Back into Self-Love

I say "back" into self-love because when you were a baby, you were all about yourself and what you needed. If you wanted something you asked for it by crying. There was no socialized interference of "It's not OK for me to ask for this, to put someone out," or questioning whether you deserved what you were asking for. You had needs and you voiced them, and the someone else came along (hopefully) and gave you what you needed. Love came from mom and dad and seemed free and unconditional.

As you moved through infancy and mom did less and less for you and you started to learn life skills and mom's support seemed to withdrawal a bit so that you could grow on your own. Later on, well-meaning parents started to teach you about life, discipline, boundaries, and the word "no." Parents would punish and sometimes withdraw love and affection when you did things they didn't agree with. You may have learned that in order to have love, you had to behave in a way that others wanted and expected you to behave; otherwise, you were disciplined and the love was withdrawn.

Then came the "should's," where you learned about how you should feel as in "How could you say that to grandma? You *should* feel very bad. Shame on you." Or, "You should eat everything on your plate; there are starving children in Africa. Don't you feel bad now?" Then there were the rules regarding how you *should* behave, such as "act like a lady" and "nice girls/boys don't do that." *Should, should, should.* And we tried to adhere to those guidelines to maintain the love and affection flowing from our parents when all that time we could have been learning how to give it to ourselves. But sadly, there are few homes where that skill is taught.

So here we are as adults, having to make up the lessons we missed or didn't receive as children so that we can feel more complete in ourselves and to stop feeling the need to seek fulfillment from the outside world through things like food, drugs, shopping, or any other external source of temporary pleasure.

Girls especially are socialized to believe that their primary role in this world is to take care of others, including kids, husbands, and other family members, in addition to work responsibilities, all before we do anything for ourselves. And when we do break down and take time for "ourselves," we were taught to feel guilty for putting our "selfish" needs ahead of others. Even churches teach us to give to others first. I am not going to question the precepts of anyone's religion, however am pretty sure they didn't mean you had to put *everybody's needs* ahead of your own, and they may even be a bit biased in that area if you really think about it.

Art class costs money; healthy food can be more expensive than junk food; and taking time for us means that maybe one of our kids can't be taken to soccer practice every single day. When we make excuses like that they result in us discarding our inner needs and replacing them with food.

An Important Habit to Create

Learning how to take care of yourself will take a lifetime of practice. I won't lie; initially it may seem strange, silly, and even feel selfish to do things for yourself by putting your needs first. But you have to learn how to do this in order to truly feel whole and complete on your own and to not have to rely on others, or worse, food to take care of your needs. Learning the keys to self-love will lead you to being a more balanced more *full*-filled being, as well as someone in that state of mind that does not try to fill themselves up with food. They give themselves exactly what they truly need.

Know that you are perfectly whole and complete just as you are, and any ideas to the contrary came from outside of you and are not true. On some level you know this; it's just a matter of accepting your true nature and getting back to self-love. The exercises I have included below are designed to enable you to return to a place of feeling love for yourself and making all your daily choices from that more life-affirming place.

Meditation: Loving Yourself

The first time you do this meditation, you may have some trouble coming up with things you love about yourself and your body. Initially, you may find that you are still sifting through those old unloving concepts to rediscover the truth of how perfect you are, and that's OK. Just notice what comes up and continue to move forward. Eventually, with practice, it will become easier. The habits of not loving yourself and putting the needs of others first were created over the course of an entire lifetime. For most of you, they won't change overnight.

Now sit back and relax. Close your eyes and allow yourself to go deep inside using *the deepening process* from earlier in the book.

When you are ready, allow your mind to focus on all the things you love about yourself, all the amazing things you do, all the talents you have, all the personal qualities that are unique and special about you. Now become aware of how good of a person you are, all the positive things you do, and all the creative contributions you make to the world. Now think about your body and how truly amazing it is. Become aware of the physical traits that you most like about yourself, no matter how small they are, think of them and notice them. Think about how you can see, hear, feel, and be all at the same time and what a true miracle that is.

Now tap into the feeling of love deep inside of yourself. Give that feeling a color and breathe in that color as you allow yourself to become completely filled with the feeling of self-love as well as acceptance of your body, mind, and spirit, knowing that all is perfect.

Relax and go a little deeper, much deeper, to a place where there is a special magical light. This is the spark of creation; the part deep inside of you that created your life initially. This is also the spark that sustains your breathing and keeps your body alive. Some people would call that spark; god, spirit, or the sound of OM. Whatever, that inner spark is for you, tap into it now. Notice that spark is perfect and full of life. Allow yourself to connect to it, bask in its energy, and feel that you and your body are perfect, whole, and complete just as they are.

Once you are able to experience those feelings strongly enjoy them for a few moments, and then when you are ready, allow your eyes to drift open as you begin your day from that place, making all your daily choices from the place of self-love.

Daily Practice

Do the above meditation as often as you need to reconnect with your feelings of self-love, and practice the following habits on a daily basis in order to reinforce this feeling so it continues to grow stronger over time.

Develop a real love for your body just the way it is. This doesn't mean you don't work on making it even healthier, but when you try to change your body from a place of hating it, you create an adversarial relationship with yourself and a resistance to change develops. How hard would you work for someone you really hated? Loving your body as it is now is the same as loving yourself, flaws and all, and it's an important part of creating positive change. Every day stand in front of the mirror, smile, and tell yourself something you really like about your body that day. At first it may be a small complement like "Your hair looks really good with that new styling product," and later it may be more like "you look amazing." It gets much easier, and it will really help you develop love for yourself.

Develop respect for your personal ambitions. What are your personal goals and wishes? What do you want to create for yourself in this life? So many of us spend a lot of energy working toward helping others achieve their goals and we forget ourselves. Stop worrying so much about the kids' futures and pay more attention to your own. It may seem selfish, but your kids seeing you happy is much more valuable to them than a bit more money in the household budget.

Don't criticize yourself. Notice where you are being critical of yourself and just like you would tell one of your children to stop picking on the other, tell your mean self to "stop" when it is saying things that aren't nice or life affirming. I will discuss this more in the next chapter, but for now practice noticing and correcting yourself when you are being judgmental with yourself.

Be your own best friend. If you are sad, mad, depressed, or just lonely you don't need food—you need *you*. Learning to be your own best friend and listening to your own internal dialogue about how and why you feel a certain way is the best thing you can do for yourself and on some level it's what you most want.

Support your decisions. Learn to stick up for yourself and support your own decisions. Don't second guess every choice you make because your boyfriend/girlfriend or spouse disagrees with you. You are entitled to your feelings, and you need to support yourself when you make decisions.

Get more exercise. This isn't just for your body; its for your mind. Although exercise will improve you general health and it's been clinically proven time and time again that this is the best, easiest, and cheapest way to improve your mood is to exercise regularly. Physical activity makes your whole self feel better and happier. Even if it's just a short walk around the block, take time for at least some exercise every day.

Ask for what you need. Politely ask for a raise if you feel you deserve it. Ask for gifts from your spouse. Ask to be seated at a nicer table at the restaurant. Ask for the discount you saw advertised. They may say "no," and that's OK, but asking for more tells yourself and the world, "I love myself. I deserve the best. I am open to receive the best and this is what I would like." It's not rude to ask for more, and it doesn't make you a bad person. If you feel that way, then you were likely taught this by parents who didn't feel that they deserved more than they got. You and everyone else deserve the best of everything, but the ones that actually get it are the ones who ask for it and realize on a core level that they deserve it. You deserve it; so work on or work on developing those feelings because you deserve it.

Notice your own body language. Do you slouch and look at the ground rather than stand straight up and look people in the eye when you pass them? If you do, then work on catching yourself and remind yourself that "I am beautiful." Looking people in the eye tells both yourself and others that you are the equal of anyone around you. This more than almost anything else will help you build your confidence, which is essential for keeping the weight off for good.

Saying "no" to requests for money, time, or favors when you don't want to do something. As I said before, women especially are socialized to say "yes" to requests for help and feel guilty when they say "no". If you don't want to give or you if you feel that you're being taken advantage of, then learning to say "no" is an essential part of loving yourself. It's not selfish to let others handle their own problems; it's about taking care of you the way you are supposed to. I highly recommend reading Anne Brown's book, *Developing Your Backbone: The Science of Saying NO* in order to help with this issue. But for now, practice saying "no" to small requests even when you don't have to. This will help you get more comfortable with expressing yourself and your needs. Then gradually move up to larger and larger requests until you are able to easily say "no" to anything. Trust me on this one, developing this skill will save you a lot of future upset.

Most importantly, take care of your own health. If you haven't had your annual physical or well woman exam, call today and schedule one; as well as a dental cleaning and eye doctor appointment. Since this process is about creating optimal health, it's very important that you make your health a priority. Many women I talk to can say that they took the dog to the vet more recently than they went for a checkup. Your physical body is sacred; you must start treating it that way.

Find a new passion. Think of something you have always wanted to learn, and sign up for a class in it. In most cities, there is a community college or resource center where you can take classes in activities ranging from ballroom dancing and painting to Feng Shui and self defense. Learning and growing as a person shouldn't stop when you finish college; you should always give yourself new challenges that enliven your life and bring you joy. New passions will feed you and help you feel *full*-filled in a way that food never could.

Do nice things for yourself. Practice giving yourself gifts of love. If you want flowers or candy, don't wait for someone else to give it to you-go out and give them to yourself. Make a gift of those treats to yourself. If you have trouble thinking of what you should do for you, try to begin by thinking about what you would want a girlfriend/boyfriend or spouse to give you and start there. When we are taking care of ourselves, it shows others how we expect to be treated, and they will respond to this example. Practice self-love by taking yourself out on dates. At first it may seem awkward to go to a movie by yourself however, it is far better than staying home and eating because you feel like you can't go out unless someone invites you. Self-love is about taking care of your wants and needs.

Exercise: Resistance

For the next few days as you practice all the processes of loving yourself, notice any mental resistances that you might come up against, become aware of what you feel when you try to do these things, and what negative words pop up in your head. Pay attention to those words and write them down. Many people often feel intense guilt about taking care of their needs. They are often overwhelmed by the feeling that it is selfish and wrong to take care of their own needs ahead of those around them. Whatever form these feelings take for you, be sure to note them and pay particular attention to whether these ideas came from you or from someone outside yourself, like a family member. Very likely these ideas came from another and over time they've become deeply ingrained in your way of life.

When these feelings come up allow them to be, but keep reminding yourself that the more you can love yourself the more you will have to share with the world. Also remember that you are an important part of the universe, and it's your responsibility to give yourself all the care you need.

Meditation: Resistance to Loving Yourself

Allow yourself to get comfortable. Focus your attention inside and fully relax into the space you are sitting or lying on, feeling completely supported in this space. Use *the deepening process* from earlier in the book to go deeper inside.

See yourself walking into a beautiful inner sanctuary. It's a quiet place of peace, a place where you go to make changes and important decisions. You may imagine a church, temple or even a library, wherever you feel most nurtured. You notice that in the center of the building there is a fire pit with a large fire burning. This fire warms your skin and brings you comfort.

As you stand or sit by the fire enjoying its warm glow, think about all the resistances and feelings that come up around the idea of loving and caring for yourself. Notice if those feelings or thoughts came from you or from someone else. Also observe whether those feelings reside in a specific part of the body or if they are only in the mind. Pay special attention to any feelings of guilt, knowing that those feelings in particular were handed to you from outside the body. Wherever they are residing now, visualize those feelings as attached to a string and begin to pull those feelings out. You no longer need them. Just pull them out of your body and throw them into the fire and allow that fire to destroy those feelings. Now notice if there are any words associated with those feelings, words about what you *should* be doing or how you *should* behave. Toss those words in the fire and feel those words leaving your body and mind, opening space for something else to come in.

Now think about any resistance you might have to *doing* things for yourself, like doing fun activities by yourself or buying yourself flowers. Observe any resistances you might feel and see yourself repeating the process of pulling those feelings out of the body and tossing them into the fire, thus ridding your body and mind of any ideas about why you shouldn't do those things. Again, pay special attention to any feelings of guilt and let that go of them.

Since you have now created more space to feel what you want to feel, allow your body and mind to fill with feelings of love and acceptance for you and all that you are. Allow yourself to really feel those feelings as you now think about all the great things you would like to do for and with yourself now that you are free of any resistances that hold you back. Once you have really tapped into those feelings of self-love and have some ideas about what you would like to do, open your eyes and begin to figure out how you are going to bring those new habits and activities into your life.

Summary

Self-love may be a skill that you have to learn after a lifetime of being told that it's "selfish," but really taking it on self-love will make every aspect of your life easier. Self-love is absolutely essential for accomplishing any goals that you have for yourself, most especially creating optimal health.

Lesson 18: Your Words Have Power—Choose Them Wisely

The Power of Words

One of the most important techniques for generating more self-love is to say loving words to yourself. We worked on this a little bit in the first lesson but it's so important that we will work on it at a deeper level in this lesson. You may not have noticed this before, but words are almost always floating around in your head. Right now that voice is probably saying to you, "What words?" This is about the words that are floating around inside your head at this point. Some words your inner voice says are supportive and kind, almost like an inner coach, while others are very critical. The latter are often demeaning and demoralizing making you feel very bad about yourself especially when you try something outside of your usual comfort zone. If you are someone who meditates, then you have probably become acutely aware of these words since this is what you try to slow down in order to reach the meditative state.

Where did those words come from? That's a complex question, but if you really listen to the words you may notice that, even though the voice is usually your own, a lot of the words sound like they come from your family. The criticisms and stern directives that your parents used to say either to you or to others in your household. From a psychological perspective, a lot of these words come from your unconscious mind, and if you pay attention you may notice that they come from different parts of your personality. For example, that part of you that wants to lose weight might say how great it would be to work out today and how great we'll feel when we get to our swimsuit weight. Meanwhile, the part of your personality that doesn't want to lose weight might say how great a Twinkie or 2, or 10 sounds and how "you can always work out tomorrow."

Most people don't realize this but unsupportive self-talk is a learned behavior you probably initially picked up from your family. If you grew up in a family that was very negative, critical, or unsupportive of each other, you may have internalized this manner of talking to yourself when you want something. If you were undervalued as a child your internal self may have taken this on as the truth and imitated your family's way of being because you internal self hadn't learned any other ways of being. If you didn't have a loving and supportive family that encouraged you and taught you how to encourage yourself to achieve all that you want in life, then your inner words will probably not be supportive and kind since you never learned to speak to yourself that way. Now your inner-self is often even more critical and judgmental than your family ever was.

Oftentimes we do not notice these negative words because they have always been there and they have a great impact on your life and your ability to achieve all your goals. Imagine if a negative person walked around with you all day telling you that you can't do this, or that, or how stupid or bad you are, or how it's dumb to even try whatever you are working on. Negative and unsupportive self-talk can make you feel like you are the biggest failure that ever lived and that you don't deserve to be happy. How could you succeed at something as difficult as losing weight with your inner voice telling you it's stupid to even try?

I once had a client who had been doing well on her new eating plan all week and then something bad happened at her office which resulted in her losing a good paying client. She got so upset that she drove straight to the drive-thru at a fast food restaurant and ordered something big, meaty, and very bad for her. She told me that the whole time she was in line at the drive-thru she heard her Mom's voice in her head telling her she was "trash," "a complete failure," and "totally worthless." This led her to add a milkshake to her already awful order of a "double burger, fries, and, oh yes, please oversize me." She ate the food in the parking lot, without even tasting it, and cried the whole way home. Does any of this sound familiar? Have you done this before too? Everyone who struggles with their weight probably has done this at one point, but in order to change our habits, we have to stop those old behaviors and do things differently.

I asked her to imagine how things would have been different if, while she was in line at the drive-thru her mind told her "Don't worry about it. We'll make it right with your client. It's OK. That's part of doing business. It happens to everyone. Why don't we go to the beach for a few minutes and walk it off?" She said if those had been the words she heard, she probably would have ordered an iced tea instead and taken a walk on the beach.

Sometimes we recycle words from other completely unrelated situations in our lives and bring them into our new endeavors. Imagine that you are a young child doing something you aren't supposed to be doing, like writing on the wall with a crayon, and your mom catches you and yells at you to stop doing that. "You are bad! Stop that! You are driving me crazy!" The words may not be the same, but the tone and theme are "You did _____. Now you are bad." Many of you are trying to control your eating in the same way: "You ate this, weigh that, and look like this—now you are bad!" This type of negative dialogue only makes you feel worse about yourself and drives you to eat more food.

After I started my most recent and only successful, attempt to lose weight, I began paying a great deal of attention to those words, and I heard some really ugly things. For instance, for every tool I bought in order to help me lose weight (book, exercise equipment, vitamin) I heard my mom's voice say, "You can't afford to spend the money on that..." I also heard my dad's voice say, "It's good that you are losing weight. Maybe you can get yourself a good husband now," and my grandmother's voice saying, "You need to lose weight so you won't look so sloppy." To my grandmother, a former beauty queen, appearance was of upmost importance. When I paid attention and became aware of what these voices were saying, I realized it would be very hard to lose weight with all that negative chatter going on in my head.

Making the Words More Supportive

How do you make the words more supportive? This may sound counterintuitive, but you can't change them by trying; that will just drive you nuts. Instead, you have to catch yourself while you're thinking an unsupportive thought, and then correct in much the same way you might argue with someone who told you something wrong. Imagine if someone called you stupid, and instead of just taking it, feeling bad, and moving on you calmly turned around and said, "No I'm not, but thanks for your concern." After a while, this person would probably no longer say that to you because you didn't accept it. This is such an important issue that I am offering several different solutions because, as you go along you will find that not every strategy will work all the time.

T. Harv Ecker, who wrote the book, *Secrets of the Millionaire Mind,* put it best in one of his seminars when he said, "You have to say to that inner voice, 'Thank you for sharing, but the truth is....'" And he is absolutely right! To this day, I use his approach for every occasional stray negative thought that arises, by telling myself something about just how wonderful and perfect I am by virtue of being myself.

Don't try to censor every word that pops into your head; you wouldn't be able to do anything else all day long, and it's not necessary. But over time, your mind can be retrained to say more positive words and you will notice fewer and fewer unsupportive thoughts if you stay on top of it. To start, I recommend trying to catch yourself thinking unsupportive thoughts several times every day or simply paying attention to the most unsupportive phrases that you say to yourself. As you correct yourself and give that voice other words to use, the messages will begin to change. You are teaching that voice how to be your inner coach and telling it how you want to be coached. And if you never had an example of someone saying supportive loving things to you in your own life, showing yourself how to support what you are doing is the best way you can create it.

Exercise, Part 1: Noticing Negative Words

Since you cannot fix a problem unless you fully understand, for the next few days spend some time noticing the words you say to yourself. Notice if there is a theme, like being critical or mean, and then See if you can determine whether the words are in your own voice or in someone else's, like your mother's. Are the ghosts of other peoples' past criticism trying to interfere with your success? Is it possible these words are trying to help you, but instead they end up sabotaging your efforts?

Make a list of the common phases or words that you hear the most (we will use this list in a later exercise). It's important that you create this list without being judgmental about what you are saying to yourself. Right now, this is just about observing and understanding this problem so that you can work out a solution to it.

When you notice that the words originally came from someone else, remember that this is not about throwing them back in their face. It's about acknowledging the truths from your childhood, even the ugly ones, so that you can realize that the formation of these negative words was not really your fault.

Part 2: Changing Negative Words

For the next part of this exercise, take out the list of words and phrases from Part 1 and after each word or phrase write an opposite truth. Here's an example:

> *"I am so fat and ugly."* The truth is "I am perfect just as I am."

> *"This will never work it never does."* The truth is "That was yesterday, this is today, and I am doing exactly what I need to do."

Once you feel that you have a good complete list, do the following meditation in order to help you release some of those old phrases and to bring in more positive ones.

Meditation: Healing Negative Words

Get into a comfortable state and allow your mind to drift deep inside. Use *the deepening process* from earlier in the book to relax more deeply.

When you are ready, picture yourself sitting on a beautiful beach. Feel the sand beneath your body, smell the salty sea air, and feel a gentle breeze on your body; making the picture as real as possible. Now think of all the negative, mean, untrue words that you or others have said about you and about your weight over the years. Use a stick to write those words in the sand. As you write them in the sand feel them leave your body and sink into the sand, as though it is able to absorb the words from your body. Keep taking the words out of your head and putting them into the sand, writing and writing until you have gotten all of those mean and untrue ones out of your mind and into the sand.

Now visualize a giant wave coming toward you on the beach, and as you step away from the water, see the wave wash over the words and erase them as though they were never there, leaving a very clear stretch of beach for you to write new words.

Now that all the old words are gone, I want you to hear the real truths of who you are inside your mind. Phrases like "I am lovely," "I am a wonderful person, whole and perfect just as I am," "I love myself." As you hear these words, use the same stick to write them in the sand. Notice that as you write these new words and new ways of thinking about yourself, that they are also going into your mind and filling the empty space those old words left behind. See those new words and new truths as waves of positive energy coming into your mind, helping you tap into your real and positive truths. Once you feel your body and mind are fully refreshed from this new way of thinking, go ahead and open your eyes.

Summary

It took me several months to work on changing my words, and in that time something magical happened: the words became more supportive with less and less effort. Now I rarely hear anything mean or unsupportive about any of the issues in my life, and that has really helped me feel better about myself.

Change doesn't happen overnight, but I can assure you I can assure you if you take this on and practice it, you will begin notice a profound difference in the way that voice speaks to you and how much success you can have with it. I went from spending all day hearing a destructive monologue about how I could never do anything right to hearing mostly loving and supportive words. In fact, when the old unsupportive language does creep in, it stands out because it happens so rarely. And for me, that is a huge miracle that has really improved the quality of my life.

Lesson 19: Acceptance vs. Giving up

I hear a lot of questions about the last 10 pounds. Those seem to be the hardest and most frustrating to lose, and the first to come back later. It's common to achieve the first 80% of your weight-loss goal relatively quickly, and then to spend almost as much time on the last 20%, all the while not really celebrating your weight loss because you aren't "perfect" yet. Sometimes very healthy, physically fit, and active women try so hard to have the body of the swimsuit model in a magazine that they totally miss how amazing they just as they are.

When someone takes a really long time to drop the last 10 pounds, it's often because they didn't have a realistic goal to begin with, both physically and emotionally. Ideally, the goal would be to get your body to its most optimal state of health, and in the meantime to learn to love your body just as it is. This will help you to avoid taking increasingly drastic weight loss methods out of frustration with no real health benefit in order to lose the last 10 pounds.

The longer you let yourself wallow in frustration and feel like you haven't accomplished your goal, the more likely you are to just give up and say, "Why should I try so hard when I am not going to reach my goal anyway? I might as well eat what I want." What's more, by continuing to feel that you have not reached your goal, you are sending a message to yourself on an unconscious level that you aren't good enough just as you are. After a while of beating yourself up like that, you'll start to feel very discouraged and possibly end up giving up on being healthy altogether, thus returning to old habits and losing all the ground you had gained.

I can attest to this as this was a major problem for me. I lost the first 70 pounds in about six months and then spent the next year trying to get down to what I thought was my ideal weight, when in reality, I was probably already sitting on what was the most ideal weight for me. Later, as the result of an illness, I did lose the last 10 pounds and became a size 6 only to discover that size didn't really suit me. My hip bones stuck out and I didn't really look very attractive in a bikini. Family and friends commented that I actually looked too thin and perhaps it was time to stop, which I did, but not really by choice. I didn't stay at that weight very long because my body wasn't able to maintain being that size, and I bounced back to the weight and size I have maintained for the past five years. My weight fluctuates a bit but stays in the same five-pound range. I am currently a size 10, a size that seems to suit my body and has been easy to maintain.

When you start the journey of weight loss, you may want it to end at a certain place, but until you shed most of the weight you hope to, it's difficult to know exactly where the end should be. Sometimes your body tells you when you are done, and it's best to allow yourself to listen. Finishing differently than you expected is not failing and its not giving up; it's about respecting your body and what it feels. Love yourself and your body enough to listen to what it wants and be happy with the outcome that's most healthy for you. Accepting what is best is the best way to avoid giving up.

Exercise: The Last 10 Pounds

If you have been sitting at your "almost there" weight for six months and are starting to feel frustrated, try asking yourself the following questions:

What do I think losing the last 10 pounds will give me that I don't have now?

If your answer has anything to with looking like a model or thinking that men will find you more attractive, consider the following: as mentioned previously, survey after survey has shown that the number one most attractive quality a woman can possess is confidence, not a size 6 body—confidence. A woman who feels good about herself no matter how much she weighs will almost always appear more attractive to most men—at least the ones you would want to date anyway—than a super skinny woman who does not feel she is attractive.

If your goal is to look perfect in a bikini, I want you to go to the beach or pool and really look at all the people there. With few exceptions (very few), nobody looks perfect in a bathing suit. It's all about being confident, holding your head high, and putting yourself out there, flaws and all. Those are the people who really enjoy themselves.

If it's anything else, I want you to ask another question:

Is there any other way I can meet the need that I am trying to meet by losing 10 more pounds?

I bet there is, and if there isn't you should still consider letting it go, unless working toward that goal brings you genuine joy.

Summary

The bottom line is that there is no shame in accepting that you've completed your journey at 150 pounds rather than 140. You are not giving up; you are accepting and congratulating yourself for a job well done and saying, "This is my body now and I am so proud." Often when you do give up the struggle something magical happens: you end up losing those last 10 pounds without even really trying.

Lesson 20: Final Success Tips

When Life Hits You in a Bad Way

Life happens in a bad way sometimes, and there is nothing you can do about it. It's easy to feel sorry for yourself when things aren't going well and to use that as an excuse to drive past the gym on the way to the drive-thru: "Yes, please supersize me, after all it's been a bad day, week, month, year" ect. There will always be things in your life that won't be as you would ideally like them to be, and food will *never* make them better, and you know it. If you want to change you can't perpetuate the habit of allowing those things to interfere with your goals in this area of your life because then they will interfere in all other areas. Life changes happen because you make a choice. You choose to either focus on being healthy and having the life you want, or letting things, often little things, derail your goals. You cannot change how life happens to you, good or bad, but you can change how you respond to it.

Thin people mostly eat the same whether they are amid chaos or calm. While it is easier to maintain a plan in the calm parts of life, the true test is to maintain this plan during a storm. If you have put yourself on a diet that is so complicated or difficult to follow that you can't maintain it when things get out of control then you have three options to choose from: 1) rethink the plan you have and dumb it down so that it's very easy for you to follow 2) choose a different eating plan, one that is so simple that you can do it no matter what, like just eating less; or 3) re-evaluate your commitment level and make a choice to ____. You can choose to allow your kids, problems at work, financial troubles, relationship troubles, or even car troubles to become excuses for you to stop using all your tools and to give up on your dreams, or you can just allow all those issues (which by the way, will never completely go away) to be there throughout your weight loss process and stick to it anyway.

It may seem easier to give up and say, "There are just so many more important things going on right now than me thinking about eating healthy. I am going to just do what I want." However, in this case "doing what you want" means falling back on old ways and perpetuating the problem. The key to getting through when life gets tough, and believe me it will at times, is to create a new habit of not letting your personal health and well-being slide when you are in crisis.

Think of it as life testing you; "How bad do you want it?" Yes, it's difficult to resist the temptation the first couple of times to chuck it all and think, "I will lose weight next month, instead." If you don't give up and stick with your new healthy habits, next month will come around, and the crisis will be over, and you will now be thinner, happier, and feel that you are in better control of yourself.

Love yourself, heal, and never give up even if you fall splat on your face (which we all do   sometimes). There is always tomorrow.

Focus on What You Want

One really important thing I've learned over the course of my life is that if you want something specific, like becoming your most healthy self, you need to focus on having or being that rather than focusing on what you aren't. Here are some good strategies to support you in that endeavor:

- Focus on and celebrate the times you stayed on your eating plan, went to your workout, or used your tools to work through an emotional issue rather than eating.
- Focus on improving your health rather than the number on the scale.
- Focus on all the great things your body can do rather than what it can't.
- Focus on the goals you are going to achieve rather than the things you didn't achieve.
- Focus on being happy about the positive changes rather than wishing for something that isn't possibly further down the road.

- Most importantly, focus on the things you love about you and what you love about your body rather than the weight you haven't lost. Even if you have to fake it, if you spend time focusing on loving your thighs then eventually you really will.

New Clothes—Not so Fast!

Most of my clients tell me their main goal is to feel more comfortable in their clothes and be able to wear a smaller size. Let's face it-there are a lot more nice clothing choices in a size 10 than a size 22. I often hear, "I just want my clothes to fit better. I want things to be looser." Those same clients are usually the first to run out to the store and buy new clothes when they drop a few pounds, and then they call me the next week extremely excited: "My pants were loose so I *had to* get some new ones." But unfortunately the new clothes are just as tight, or tighter, than the old ones were when they started this process. This invariably triggers the whole drama of feeling fat and bad about themselves all over again, which often makes them want to emotionally eat in order to feel better.

My advice is to savor your victory for as long as possible. Wear those loose jeans, baggy shirts, and ill-fitting skirts as long as you can without looking like you have a problem. Here's the thing, when you are sitting there in loose pants, you are seeing and most importantly, feeling the results of your efforts. Those feelings are a great motivator for staying with your program. Loose pants don't inspire you to fill them; they are showing you that what you are doing is working.

Celebrate Your Victories in a Big Way

Life victories are cause for real celebration, and losing all the weight definitely qualifies as a major victory. Celebrating your victories is an essential part of keeping yourself motivated on this journey. No matter how much weight you have to lose, the process is likely to take at least several months, so I always tell people that they need to plan some kind of meaningful celebration every 10 pounds or so.

However, the key to these celebrations is that they cannot be centered on food. Food can be a part of the event, but it can't be the glue that brings that event together. You don't want to celebrate losing 10 pounds by going to Baskin Robbins, because, not only is that inappropriate, but you want to learn how to get into the habit of celebrating your victories without food. It's OK to have a picnic with food, as long as the focus is about enjoying time with yourself or celebrating with others and being outside. I once celebrated by going rock-climbing with friends, other times we went camping, and once we even went bowling. But my biggest, most outrageous celebration came at the end.

My boyfriend at the time suggested that I celebrate reaching my goal by baring it all at the local nude beach. At first I said "no" because, well, that just sounded nuts. But then I realized how appropriate it would be. Having been overweight since I was 12, I was always very self-conscious about my body, and even though I lived within five miles of the beach, I rarely went for a swim because I felt embarrassed. Doing the Full Monty at a nude beach seemed like a good way to get comfortable with myself around others doing the same. Taking all my clothes off and being free in a physical way really represented my emotional transformation as well. I was finally free.

Of course you don't need to do anything that outrageous—I probably won't do it again. But, I am really glad that I did it because that experience really meant something to me in a way that dinner out never could.

Train for Something

If you want to take your process of creating optimal health to a higher level, I recommend challenging yourself to an even greater degree by signing up for something really hard like a marathon, triathlon, or bike race. Preparing for events like these requires a huge time commitment and dedication to long-term training, but the payoff goes beyond just the physical changes your body goes through. The process of pushing your body to do something beyond what you would normally think of yourself being capable of gives you an amazing sense of accomplishment and helps you feel on a core level how truly powerful you are.

About a year after I lost all the weight, my father invited me to do a one-day family hike up Mount Whitney in California, a 22-mile hike with a 6,100 elevation gain. This hike would be strenuous because of its elevation and length, and would require several months of training; even with that I still wasn't sure I was physically capable of doing it. I decided to try it anyway because, in addition to it being a very beautiful hike, I was also hoping for a bonding experience with my dad, a person I did not have a very deep connection with. He helped me make it to the top by carrying my pack for the last mile when I was ready to give up. That shared experience helped to repair a badly damaged relationship and to create the new, happier connection that we have today. The experience also made me physically and emotionally stronger, and I can't fully describe how amazing that feels. I can honestly say that was the hardest thing I have ever done, and it broadened the horizons of what I thought I could achieve. It made me realize that if I can do that, I truly can do anything.

Clients and friends who have trained for and completed a marathon describe many of the same feelings I had: the sense of accomplishment and the feeling on a very core level that they are capable of so much more than they thought possible. In addition, the sense of bonding and being with other people who have had similar experiences feels amazing. I would highly recommend the experience of pushing yourself in this way to anyone.

If it's something you are interested in, there are meet-up groups (meetup.com) in almost every city where people can connect with others who are also training for something. Joining one of these groups will help you train even before the event happens. I used meetup.com and outdoorsclub.org to connect with fellow hikers who were also training to hike Mount Whitney.

Your Egg

When I was in high school, one of the things we had to do in human biology class, also known as Sex Ed, was to carry around a raw egg. This raw egg was supposed to represent the baby you might create if you had unprotected sex, and it was meant to show you much focus and responsibility this very important thing would require.

You couldn't throw it in your locker and forget about it, or mistreat it in any way; you had to care for this thing for the whole week and make it your number one priority. Although this exercise taught me to hate raw eggs, it did show me how much effort and thought goes into taking care of something that is really important.

Creating lifelong optimal health is a lot like that too. You don't just start, give up, forget about it, and then expect results. This has to be something you nurture, take responsibility for, commit to, take with you everywhere you go, and make it part of your life. You have to become that vision of your dream person by letting go of the fat person you used to be and by nurturing your inner thin person that is growing stronger inside of you now.

You can do this by keeping this vision with you at all times, no matter what happens or how you slip up, and you will slip up sometimes, but it's part of the process. You can also do this by being flexible and a bit introspective about your journey so that when things don't go according to plan, you can ask yourself "Why?" and then adjust your vision according to your changing needs and ideas.

You don't have to spend all your time on this project, but you do need to commit 100% to your vision. The means of getting there can and should change along the way, but the final vision (ultimate goal) of what you want to create for yourself should remain the same.

Exercise: A Constant Reminder of Ideal Health

Choose something small that represents what reaching your ideal weight means to you. This could be a picture, a special rock that reminds you of the beach, or something entirely different. What's important is that is means "ideal health" to you and that you can take it with you. I want you put this object where you will see it frequently so that it can remind you of your commitment to yourself and to this process.

Final Thoughts

The view from the other end of that long path to creating optimal health for yourself is amazing, but it's always a work in progress, even after you reach your goals. Making your body as healthy as it can be is truly the ultimate act of self-love and self-respect. It's the greatest gift you can give yourself.

I know that it's possible for everyone to be the healthiest version of themselves, even if that ends up looking different than you thought it would—a size 10 rather than a size 2. But whatever that looks like for you, love yourself enough to do all you can to create as much health as possible no matter what size you are.

When I was a child, I had a plaque on my wall that read: "Do not go where the path may lead. Go instead where there is no path and leave a trail." This book was my trail, and I hope it helps to lead you to your highest goals— I look forward to seeing you there.